A
Woman's
Book
of
Meditation

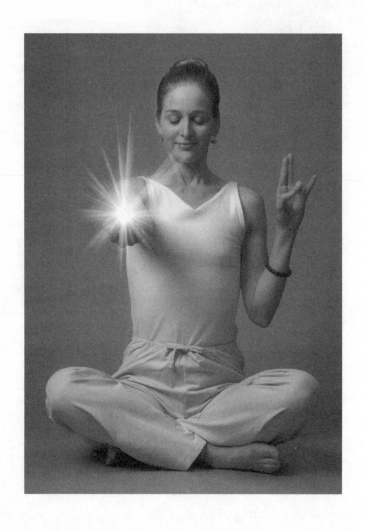

Foreword by Michael McGee, M.D.

PHOTOGRAPHS BY RALPH MERCER

Avery
a member of
Penguin Group (USA) Inc.
New York

A
Woman's
Book
of
Meditation

Discovering the Power
of a Peaceful Mind

HARI KAUR KHALSA

Published by the Penguin Group
Penguin Group (USA) Inc., 375 Hudson Street, New York, New York 10014, USA • Penguin Group
(Canada), 90 Eglinton Avenue East, Suite 700, Toronto, Ontario M4P 2Y3, Canada
(a division of Pearson Penguin Canada Inc.) • Penguin Books Ltd, 80 Strand, London WC2R 0RL,
England • Penguin Ireland, 25 St Stephen's Green, Dublin 2, Ireland (a division of Penguin Books
Ltd) • Penguin Group (Australia), 250 Camberwell Road, Camberwell, Victoria 3124, Australia
(a division of Pearson Australia Group Pty Ltd) • Penguin Books India Pvt Ltd, 11 Community Centre,
Panchsheel Park, New Delhi–110 017, India • Penguin Group (NZ), Cnr Airborne
and Rosedale Roads, Albany, Auckland 1310, New Zealand (a division of Pearson
New Zealand Ltd) • Penguin Books (South Africa) (Pty) Ltd, 24 Sturdee Avenue,
Rosebank, Johannesburg 2196, South Africa

Penguin Books Ltd, Registered Offices: 80 Strand, London WC2R 0RL, England

Most Avery books are available at special quantity discounts for bulk purchase for sales promotions, premi-
ums, fund-raising, and educational needs. Special books or book excerpts also can be created to fit specific
needs. For details, write Penguin Group (USA) Inc. Special Markets, 375 Hudson Street, New York, NY
10014.

Library of Congress Cataloging-in-Publication Data
Khalsa, Hari Kaur.
A woman's book of meditation: discovering the power of a peaceful mind/Hari Kaur Khalsa;
foreword by Michael McGee, M.D.; photography by Ralph Mercer.
p.   cm.
Includes index.
ISBN 1-58333-253-7
1. Kundalini.   2. Meditation.   3. Women—Religious life.   4. Spiritual exercises.   I. Title.
II. Title: Discovering the power of a peaceful mind.
BL1238.56.K86K525   2006   2006042792
204'.36—dc22

Printed in the United States of America
1   3   5   7   9   10   8   6   4   2

This book is printed on acid-free paper. ∞

Book design by Lee Fukui

For Yogi Bhajan
And my husband, Dave Frank

Acknowledgments

I first want to express my deep and heartfelt gratitude to Yogi Bhajan for bringing the teachings of Kundalini Yoga for women to the United States. His tireless dedication to uplifting women remains a continual inspiration to me.

This project would not be possible without the support of the editorial staff at Penguin Books. I express my gratitude and thanks to Kristen Jennings for her belief in this project and to Rebecca Behan for her support and great editing, and Anna Ghosh, my literary agent, for her support.

Thanks to the beautiful Shelly Loheed for being the model for this book; her dedication and commitment to this project and to the teachings of Kundalini Yoga and meditation radiate from every photograph. I also thank Ralph Mercer for his artistic dedication to yoga photography, stylist Paula Dion, the Kundalini Research

Institute for its commitment to sharing the teachings of Yogi Bhajan, my fellow yoga teachers and teacher trainers, and the many students who through their dedication continue to give me the opportunity to teach. Thanks to Sat Bir Singh Khalsa, research scientist at Harvard Medical School, for his knowledge of the body of scientific research as it pertains to yoga and meditation. Grateful thanks to Lea Kramer for her assistance with Sanskrit notations, Dharm for his timely research and more, Dr. Michael McGee for bridging East and West in his work with his patients and sharing this important work in the foreword of this book, Irene Frank for her open heart and open mind, and Machelle M. Seibel, M.D., for his partnership on the first book of this series, *A Woman's Book of Yoga: Embracing Our Natural Life Cycles.*

Contents

Foreword

Meditation is the foundation of all spiritual practices and traditions. What has been known throughout the ages by sages from every time and place is now the subject of scientific inquiry. We now know that meditation actually changes the brain. Neuroimaging studies show, among other things, greater overall brain-wave synchrony and increased metabolism in experienced meditators. These studies confirm that changes in states of consciousness produced by meditation correlate with changes in brain states. This exciting research holds great promise for elucidating the neuroanatomy and neurophysiology of enhanced states of consciousness. There is also a wealth of clinical research that demonstrates an association between meditation, health, and well-being.

Of course, we've always known, anecdotally, that people who meditate tend to live happier, healthier lives. The practice of giving gentle and loving attention to this present moment through contemplative, concentrative, or mindfulness techniques results in beneficial changes in consciousness and in overall health. Through meditative practices we learn to dis-identify with our time-based thoughts and feelings and instead learn to simply "Be." In this state our minds open up. We learn not to judge our experiences. We gradually understand that our thoughts and feelings alone do not define us. We begin to experience greater peace, love, and the simple joy of existence. We are more conscious of the miraculous wonder of being alive. We develop a deeper knowing, or intuition, of what is true and right for us in each moment. And as we grow in meditation we begin to act out of that deeper knowing rather than in response to what we happen to be thinking and feeling.

I personally discovered meditation when I was in medical school at Stanford University in 1979. My own practice has brought about both a change in consciousness for me and has also influenced my work with my patients. It has taught me to not take my thoughts quite so seriously and not be quite so judgmental (or at least to notice when my mind does judge!). I've gradually learned to be more present more of the time throughout the day. This gives a directness and clarity to my awareness. I've come to see the mind as a tool that I use, rather than allowing my mind to use me. My practice serves as a spring of energy that works to renew and refresh each day.

I regularly teach meditative exercises to my patients and encourage them to incorporate a meditative practice into their daily lives. I have seen countless patients benefit medically from these efforts as they gradually develop a greater sense of peace, equanimity, and perspective in their lives. Over and over again I've observed that their treatment just seems to go better when my patients make the effort to meditate on a daily basis. Often problems and conflicts just seem to dissolve away in the stillness that accompanies awareness. My patients tell me they are happier and more loving toward others—and they typically find that their health improves along with their mood. As with any major lifestyle change I recommend to my patients, the challenge lies in guiding and motivating people to develop the discipline of a regular spiritual practice. For many people, this simply goes against the grain of their busy, activity-focused lives. And that, of course, is exactly the point!

Ours is a time of great paradox. We live in a world of astounding material abundance but in a time of great peril—both consequences of the human mind. Despite our material comforts, our many pleasures, and our increased longevity, people on the whole seem no happier than they were two hundred years ago. Perhaps happiness and well-being spring from a wisdom that lies beyond and beneath the fruits of the mind, a wisdom that can only be tapped through a practice of meditation. Our culture is currently out of balance, with too much activity and not enough solitude and stillness—the ground out of which wisdom grows.

This book addresses not only meditation but the special needs of women pursuing a meditative practice. Women have special gifts and unique psychological attributes. As a rule, women are more connected than men to the experience of Being and to their emotions.

Women face special challenges as well. The hormonal shifts in a woman's body create special physical and emotional states.

Women, more often than men, face the challenge of being the primary caregiver in the family while also pursuing a career.

I have known Hari Kaur Khalsa for a number of years. Her own practice of meditation, combined with her gifts for writing and teaching, make her uniquely qualified to write this book. Here she shares with you her wisdom and the benefits of the practice that she has personally touched so many lives with.

May this book be a resource to change the lives of women looking to enhance their happiness and well-being through the practice of meditation.

Michael McGee, M.D.

Introduction

Everything depends on your mental outlook. . . . All of your experience is filtered through the creativity and appraisal of your mind. Happy and unhappy belong to your mind, not to the world. —Yogi Bhajan

Kundalini Yoga is a total practice that includes exercises and yoga postures, meditation, and deep relaxation. This book explores the powerful healing techniques of Kundalini Yoga Meditation in a format designed specifically for women. Throughout the book you will learn how to use meditation to help you develop a positive self-image and heal negative patterns of thinking and self-limiting belief systems.

Meditation practices are as old as the history of humankind. There is recorded evidence of meditation practices as early as 4,500 years ago in ancient texts of the Indian subcontinent. Meditation techniques vary from culture to culture, and include simple meditative breathing techniques with counting (as referred to by Herb Benson, M.D., as the Relaxation Response), the walking meditations of the Buddhist traditions, meditative prayer as taught in Christian and Jewish traditions, and meditation techniques involving visualization, physical postures, and specific affirmations.

As of this writing, there are more than 250 scientific studies that document the wide-ranging benefits of yoga and meditation in the lives of those who practice them. One study has concluded that regular meditation actually helps to adjust your brain chemistry— reducing stress hormones such as cortisol. When you change your blood chemistry in this way, you physiologically shift out of the fight-or-flight stress syndrome and into a more relaxed and healthy physiological state. This simple and profound proven effect of meditation can be considered a first step toward attaining deeper levels of self-realization and healing. In addition, it has been shown that regular meditation can help women manage stress more effectively and improve the quality of their communication skills and their relationships. Meditation has been scientifically demonstrated to lower blood pressure, help insomnia, strengthen the immune system, reduce anxiety, prevent aging of the brain, lower heart rate, and help reduce chronic pain.

For all of our advances in science, technology, and self-empowerment, the question I hear most from my students is "How can I live a happy life?" According to the teachings of Kundalini Yoga, the human being is a complex creation, and implicit in this complex structure is the potential to experience bliss and happiness independent of circumstances. Your happiness is within your reach! Meditation is the way.

As you'll discover, meditation is exercise for your mind. Each time you meditate, you gain a deeper understanding of the nature of your mind—how it perceives and reacts to the world around you, and how your thoughts generate desires and preferences, attitudes and opinions. When you meditate, you are cleansing your subconscious mind—the storehouse of your life experiences, and your reactions to them—so that your natural happiness and radiance can shine more brightly.

Kundalini Yoga is a unique practice. When Yogi Bhajan came to the United States from India in the late 1960s, he taught the most guarded and ancient teachings of yoga openly and tirelessly. This book is drawn from the wealth of teachings Yogi Bhajan shared with thousands of women from 1968 until his passing in 2004.

I had the fortunate opportunity to work with and learn directly from Yogi Bhajan for fourteen years. His teachings for women have touched my heart, strengthened my identity, and allowed me to feel grace in the most challenging situations. The teachings of Kundalini Yoga—the philosophy, the practices, and the lifestyle training—have given me a strong foundation that allows for deep healing and transformation. As a result of my practice, my marriage is better, my ability to withstand transitions is stronger, and my energy level is high. Perhaps most important, I feel that my foundation as a woman is built on self-respect and an unshakable core strength.

What is the purpose of life? The purpose of life is tomorrow.
What is tomorrow? Tomorrow is getting up and knowing who
you are, knowing that God is with you, and knowing you can
handle yourself with grace. —Yogi Bhajan

To me this quote embodies the foundation of these teachings. There is inspiration for tomorrow because I know who I am—my identity is clear and my mind is calm. I am confident that the reality of existence is more than what we see, and I can trust I am strong enough to handle anything that comes my way.

A Woman's Book of Meditation is both an introduction to meditation for beginning meditators and an in-depth educational tool for experienced practitioners. Beginning students of meditation can easily understand the basic benefits of meditating and learn how to begin a personal practice as described in chapters one, two, and three. More experienced practitioners (or inspired beginners!) can expand and deepen their practice by applying the concepts presented in chapter four. Scientific studies supporting the benefits of a meditation practice are discussed in chapter five.

The meditations listed in chapter six outline a lifetime of healing meditative practices for women of all ages. As you move through the natural transitions in your life, refer to this section frequently for support.

I have seen countless women benefit from the teachings of Kundalini Yoga as taught by Yogi Bhajan. It is my prayer that each woman who encounters these teachings will experience their transformative and healing power. I sincerely hope that this book will inspire you to begin a meditation practice and will serve as a useful resource for you throughout the transitions of your life.

Let's begin!

1

The Basics
of Kundalini
Meditation

Your mind can be your best friend or your worst
enemy. As an ally, your mind can organize your
world and effectively guide your actions. As an
adversary, your mind can be jumpy and unfocused, and it can easily attach to negative patterns of thinking that stem from your fears
and insecurities. Practicing meditation can help you to develop a
positive relationship with your mind and teach you how to direct
your mind's power toward the realization of your full potential.

We live in stressful times. Women are often called upon to play
many roles, and the demands on your time and energy can be extensive. Many women suffer from a syndrome of being overstressed

and overworked. Balancing a modern lifestyle with self-care can be difficult, and self-care is often neglected. Without attention to daily rejuvenation, the constant pressures of family and career can be exhausting on every level.

In addition to dealing with the daily stresses of life, your mind is bombarded by information and images that you may not have time to process. An exploitive media and society's unrealistic ideals regarding our physical bodies and the process of aging constantly confront us as women. The information age places a huge demand on our nervous systems, requiring us to keep up with all the details needed to navigate our lives. This combination of exhaustion, societal pressures, and information overload can have a negative effect on your mental state, and fuel disempowering, destructive thought patterns. These negative thought patterns can cloak your true identity of beauty and grace.

Fortunately, a woman's mind has a natural, inborn capacity to heal itself of all these types of imbalances. Meditation is the best way to tap into this limitless healing power. Meditation will open within you an inner reservoir of energy and wisdom that you can use to deal more effectively with the challenges that come your way. When a woman learns to meditate, she learns to manage her own stress by identifying troublesome thinking patterns and strengthening her nervous system. She learns how to replenish her energy and repair herself on every level. The result of a regular meditation practice is an increased ability to deal with daily life, renewed optimism and enthusiasm for living, and an expanded spiritual awareness.

The Journey of Self-Healing Through Meditation

When you begin the practice of meditation, you may have certain goals, such as achieving a more peaceful life, healing negative thought patterns, clearing the effects of life traumas, or sustaining more meaningful partnerships. As in any creative endeavor, you will inevitably experience both exhilarating breakthroughs and unexpected obstacles. Some of the obstacles you may encounter during your meditation practice are discussed later in this book—reread these sections whenever you need extra inspiration for your journey. As you continue your practice, you will notice a deeper level of transformation occurring within you. You may find that you experience these deeper levels of spiritual development through healing your memories of past negative incidents, thereby gaining a greater appreciation of the present moment. A new clarity of perception results from meditation, which will allow you to see the beauty of life more clearly and will inspire you to make better decisions. The practice of Kundalini Meditation as outlined in this book is powerful and effective. Regular practice of the meditations in this book *will* transform you and improve the quality of your life.

You can meditate anywhere, at any time. However, meditating in an environment supportive to your practice can be more enjoyable and effective. Practice meditation in a clean and clutter-free environment. If possible, set aside a room or a space in your living area that you use exclusively for meditation. You may want to create an altar to inspire your practice. On your altar, you can place pictures, quotes, books, flowers, or anything that inspires you. Design your meditation area in such a way that simply looking at your meditation space uplifts your spirit. There can be great power and beauty in a meditation area—it is a sacred place you will return to again and again for inspiration and rejuvenation.

YOGA AND RELIGION

In this book you will frequently encounter the yogic concepts of the Divine, God, Infinity, Spiritual, True Self, and other words referring to the higher realities of life. Practicing yoga and meditation is not to be confused with one's religious beliefs. Yoga is based in practices aimed at giving you an experience of the blissful part of yourself that transcends the senses and the mundane dimension of daily life. As such, there is no inherent conflict between meditation practice and any religious path. Women can practice the meditations in this book and follow any religion of their choosing.

If possible, commit to a specific time for meditation practice. Daily practice is recommended in all meditation traditions in order to experience the deeper benefits of meditation. Start with twenty minutes. If you cannot find twenty minutes each day, schedule twenty-minute sessions when you can, at least several times a week. Take the phone off the hook, and if necessary be assertive in clearing your schedule for your practice! Treat your meditation time as if it were an appointment with a client. You may find it helpful to link your meditation practice with another regular activity—for example, before breakfast, immediately upon returning from work, or before going to bed. Linking your meditation time with another activity will help you to remember and fulfill your commitment.

You may find it useful to keep a meditation diary. Your diary should include the dates of your meditation sessions and may cover any experiences that seem worthy of note. You may want to include in your diary any insights you receive while meditating, any strategies that helped you maintain your concentration during meditation, and the specific effects of your practice. Reviewing your meditation diary periodically can be a valuable tool for obtaining self-knowledge and can assist you in achieving your meditation goals.

It is best not to eat within two hours of beginning your meditation practice, so you can spend the time meditating instead of digesting! However, do not try to meditate if you are very hungry. Instead, eat a light snack of fruit or a small amount of vegetable protein to give you energy for meditation. If you eat heavy foods such as meats, fried foods, and refined sugars, your digestive system will have to work hard and long to break down the foods and absorb the nutrients while eliminating the waste. Lighter, less processed vegetarian foods can be more easily digested and the vitamins and minerals in the food can be absorbed quickly. Although meditation can be practiced irrespective of one's diet, many women will feel lighter if they eat a vegetarian diet, and a vegetarian diet may make it easier for you to concentrate.

Each meditation in this book includes the following basic five elements:

1. Seated meditation posture

2. Breathing pattern

3. Mudras—postures for your hands, arms, and body

4. Eye focus

5. Mental focus—a mantra or visualization

Let's examine these elements more closely:

How to Sit for Meditation

Meditation is an active discipline that stimulates and adjusts your nervous system and glandular system. Yoga and meditation work to stimulate the energy associated with your spinal cord, so keeping your back in an upright and lengthened posture is recommended to assist the meditation process. You can meditate seated in a chair, but if you do it is recommended, if possible, that your spine not touch the back of the chair. If you are seated on the floor, it is recommended that you do not lean against a wall. If sitting for meditation is difficult for you without support, use whatever supports you need. You may build up stronger back muscles and more leg and hip flexibility from yoga stretching or other forms of exercise.

These are the three basic seated postures for meditation practice:

Easy Pose (*Sukhasana*)

This is the most common cross-legged position. Sit on the floor and cross your legs. If you feel tension in your knees, ankles, or back, try sitting on a folded blanket or cushion. You can use the blanket or cushion each time you meditate or exercise.

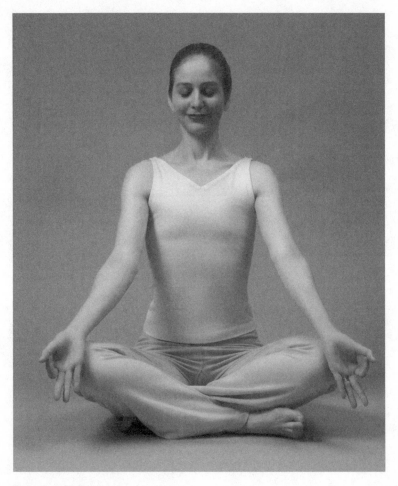

Easy Pose (*Sukhasana*)

Rock Pose (*Vajrasana*)

Sit on your heels on the floor. This is an excellent pose for women. It supports the back and stimulates digestion. Rock Pose puts pressure on and adjusts your reproductive organs. If you find Rock Pose comfortable, you can use it for any meditation.

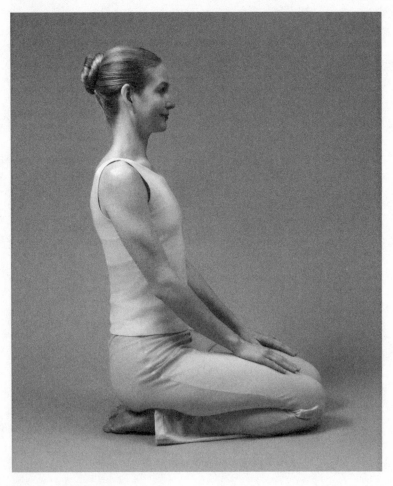

Rock Pose (*Vajrasana*)

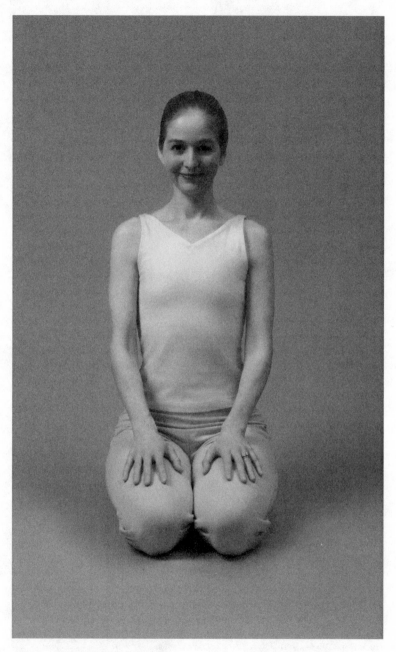

Rock Pose—(*Vajrasana*), front view

Egyptian Pose in a Chair

Sit in a chair with your feet flat on the floor. If your feet do not reach the floor, place books or a low footstool under your feet so they are flat. Lengthen your spine and hold it away from the back of the chair. Relax your hands on your thighs.

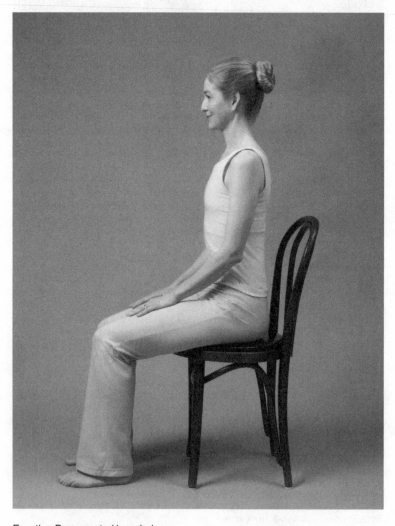

Egyptian Pose, seated in a chair

Taking the time to set your meditation posture so you can sit as comfortably as possible creates a strong foundation for your practice. When the spine is positioned correctly, you can meditate in a state of ease. You will feel as if you are perfectly balanced between effort and non-effort, or relaxation. Many students new to meditation find that sitting quietly and remaining still can be the first challenge of meditation. Feel free to adjust your posture or stretch if you need to, but also hold the intention to be still for the length of your meditation session. As you build your meditation practice, you will feel more moments of ease and of balance in mind and body. Read the descriptions of the seated poses often to refresh your memory and rejuvenate your posture.

In order to properly align your spine, you need to pay special attention to each region of the spine. The ancient texts of yoga teach that the point of energetic balance for all yoga postures is your navel point. The navel point is located about 1 to 1½ inches below your belly button. This muscular and energetic center can be considered the core for the inner resources you need to physically hold the seated meditative postures.

The yogic approach is to align the spine by contracting certain muscles that help to keep the spine lengthened and steady. These muscular contractions are called Body Locks, or bandhas. For the purposes of this book, we will concentrate on two of the bandhas called *Mula Bandha,* or Root Lock, and *Jalandhara Bandha,* or Neck Lock. These two Body Locks work together to help you maintain a steady and supported seated position; Root Lock stabilizes your lower spine to relieve lower back stiffness and support your torso, and Neck Lock lengthens your upper spine and neck so you can maintain the natural curve in your cervical spine, avoiding neck tension, breath obstruction, and upper back stiffness.

Root Lock (*Mula Bandha*)

The Root Lock helps strengthen the muscles of your lower back and is the foundation of all yoga poses and all seated meditation postures. The application of Root Lock will help you maintain the seated postures by aligning your lower spine so you can sit without any additional stress to your lower back.

To apply Root Lock, you are instructed to sequentially contract the muscles of the anus, and while holding that contraction, contract the pelvic muscles as though you are stopping the flow of urine. Holding these contractions, pull in and up on the navel point. With practice, these contractions become less like squeezing particular muscles and more like stabilizing your pelvic floor and lower spine. The practice of Root Lock can help you strengthen your pelvic floor (quite beneficial for women throughout life) and protect your lower back from the stresses of improper posture. Many women are familiar with Kegel exercises, pelvic strengthening exercises recommended for women during and after pregnancy and at menopause to strengthen their pelvic muscles. Root Lock is similar to Kegel exercises but includes a slight contraction of the lower abdominal muscles as well. Some meditations may instruct you to apply Root Lock at the end as you suspend your breath. This combination helps to create a Still Point, a moment of stillness that consolidates the benefits of the meditation and allows you to experience your meditative mind more easily. Lightly applying Root Lock during meditation may help you stay energized by stimulating the navel point for increased energy and stabilizing your posture for endurance.

· · ·

Note: Persons with high blood pressure, vertigo, high intercranial pressure, or amenorrhea should not practice Root Lock. Do not practice Root Lock if you are pregnant or on the first day of your menstrual cycle. If you are not sure whether this practice is appropriate for you, consult your physician.

Neck Lock (*Jalandhar Bandh*)

Neck Lock is a position of the neck, head, and chest that supports proper alignment. When you apply this lock, you are assuring that your neck is positioned to hold the weight of your head without straining the spine. It is common for people to strain their necks by collapsing the back of the neck and holding the chin high. This can be the result of extended periods of sitting with improper posture and can become a habit. By applying Neck Lock you can help to lengthen your spine and thus allow your breath to flow freely and energy to circulate evenly throughout your spine. Both the Root Lock and Neck Lock are important elements of ideal seated posture for meditation or any other seated activity.

To apply Neck Lock, first apply a mild Root Lock, pulling your navel point toward your spine. Then lift your chest. The more flexibility you have in your back, the more easily you can lift your chest and apply the Neck Lock. Many people are quite tense between the shoulder blades, so you may need to loosen up your upper back before you meditate and apply the Neck Lock so you can sit more easily. Next, pull your chin in (not down) to straighten the natural backward curve of your neck. As your chest lifts, allow your shoulder blades to drop down so that you can avoid hunching your shoulders and rounding your upper back.

·   ·   ·

Note: Refer to the suggested warm-up exercises to help you apply Root Lock and Neck Lock so you can feel more comfortable during seated meditation.

Meditation and Your Breath

In all meditation traditions, the awareness and regulation of one's breath is an important element of practice. And while mind, identity, and consciousness may be abstract terms for some women, breath is a physical reality for all. Through the practice of breathing techniques and the focusing of your attention on your breath, you can learn to direct your energy and your thoughts. The science of directing your energy through breathing practices is called *pranayama*. Kundalini Yoga meditations make use of many kinds of breathing techniques that have particular effects on your mental state and body chemistry.

Both your breath rate and the depth of your breath can be considered indicators of your mental and physiological states. Deeper, slower breathing is a sign of a more relaxed and meditative mind, while shallow and more frequent breathing can be an indication of stress or excitement, or an overemphasis on the positive or negative minds (see chapter three). Practicing the *pranayama* techniques in this book will teach you to quickly shift your mental and/or emotional state and help you feel more relaxed. It really works!

The breath is valued in meditation as the energy of life itself. By regulating your breath you can manage your life energy, or *prana,* and increase your awareness and sensitivity. If you have a consistent awareness and true appreciation and gratitude for your breath, you can be more appreciative of the gift of life.

Breaking the Habit of Strained Breathing—
Long Deep Yogic Breathing

As a result of stress and improper posture, many people do not breathe deeply or efficiently. When you take a deep breath, ideally your ribs should expand as your shoulders stay steady and relaxed. When you inhale, at times you may feel your shoulders lift and your neck compress. This is an indication that you are breathing ineffectively.

In order to help you break the habit of strained breathing, practice abdominal breathing. Lie on your back and place your hand on your belly. As you inhale, allow your abdominal area to expand, then expand your rib cage area, and, finally, expand your upper chest. This motion will help you train your diaphragm muscles to flatten as you inhale and allow your lungs to expand, thus allowing you to take a deep breath. As you exhale, allow your upper chest, rib cage area, and abdominal area to relax toward your spine. Practice the Long Deep Yogic Breath like this until it feels comfortable and natural. Long Deep Breathing is done primarily through your nose. This breath warms, humidifies, and filters the air entering your lungs; you are delivering the highest quality air to your lungs in the most efficient manner. Breathing consciously through your nose instead of your mouth will slow your breath rate, which allows for higher awareness and a more relaxed state.

As you practice yoga meditation, this will become the natural way you breathe all the time. Watch any young child and you will understand how natural long deep breathing is. However, as we age, stress often tightens up the belly, which causes us to get into the habit of breathing using the large chest muscles. Breathing correctly gives your body a precious gift. Practice slow long deep breathing, and enjoy its many benefits!

All breathing techniques should be practiced with attention and ease. Make sure not to strain your breathing in any way. Here are a few basic breathing techniques you will encounter throughout this book:

Segmented Breathing

Segmented breathing is a technique to refine your breath and manage your moods. Take a few Long Deep Yogic Breaths first. Sit straight in a chair or sit comfortably cross-legged (Easy Pose, page 7) on a flat surface. You can practice this as you lie on your back while you are learning. As you inhale, break your breath into 4 equal segments (sniffs). Hold this breath in for a few seconds. Then exhale, breaking the breath again into 4 equal segments (sniffs). Hold that breath out for a few seconds. Continue inhaling in 4 equal segments and exhaling in 4 equal segments. It may take you a little while to make each segment equal and have a complete inhale and exhale. Next, inhale in 4 equal segments and exhale one long continuous breath. Repeat this pattern a few times and feel the difference. This 4/4 breath is primarily used for relaxation—it is very effective in working with emotional and mental states. It also will help increase your strength, vitality, and mental focus. Segmented breathing is a yogic secret. Once you learn it, you will have a useful tool for managing your moods.

Suspending Your Breath (Antara Kumbhaka)

You can affect your autonomic nervous system by consciously changing your breath rate. Changing your breath rate will bring about a shift in your physiological and mental state. A normal breath rate is about 20 breaths per minute. During yoga practice, when you bring the breath down to 8 breaths per minute, you will automatically enter a meditative state.

At the end of many exercises, you will be instructed to suspend your breath briefly before you relax. Suspending your breath is like holding your breath, but without the strain or tension you normally feel in your chest or shoulders. This process stimulates your experience of the Still Point (as described on page 12), a basic goal of yoga and meditation.

To suspend your breath, inhale and retain your breath, keeping your chest expanded. If you feel any tension, let some breath out and try again. Remember to feel relaxed, even as you retain your breath. Relax your shoulders back and focus your eyes at your Brow Point, between your eyebrows and at the top of your nose. Become still and feel light and open. Hold your concentration gently at the brow in stillness. (This concentration is discussed in greater detail on page 18.) Suspending your breath after the physical experience of the exercises and the repetition of mantras, you will experience the Still Point. This stillness is in contrast to the movements just completed; it is this contrast that allows you to enter the meditative, quiet state of mind. And this experience of stillness will become deeper when you apply the Root Lock, described on page 12.

Mudras—Energetic Seals for Effective Meditation

Some meditations include specific hand or arm postures (seals) and positions or movements. The arm and hand postures, called mudras, are considered energetic seals. Each seal stimulates energy in your body to circulate in particular patterns, creating a healing state for your body and mind. In order to understand the science of mudra, consider how subtle and yet effective body language can be. Consider how some gestures are welcoming, some defensive, and still others elegant and beautiful. Consider the importance of fine motor control as an indicator of brain health and activity. Consider how universal some movements are, such as placing your hands over your heart for love and devotion, throwing your arms up in the air for celebration, or opening your arms to receive or give a hug.

Some mudras will help you calm your emotions; others can help give you energy and balance. Over time you will develop the sensitivity to appreciate the effects of these elegant and subtle body postures.

Eye Focus During Meditation

Most meditations will instruct you to focus your eyes in a particular way. The following eye focus points are the most common:

The Third Eye Point (*Shambavi Mudra*)

This eye focus is also often called the Brow Point Focus. The Brow Point is located at the top of your nose, between your eyebrows and at the location of your pituitary gland. To focus your eyes in this way, bring your attention to the Brow Point with your eyes gently raised. The Third Eye Point focus stimulates your pituitary gland and triggers the opening of your intuitive faculties.

The Lotus Point (*Agiaa Chakra Bandh*)

The Lotus Point is located at the bottom tip of your nose, and this eye focus is referred to as the Lotus Point Focus. Meditating with your eyes focused at the tip of your nose can help you control your mind. This focus can be done with the eyes open, closed, or partially closed. When you focus your eyes in this way, you will stimulate the frontal lobe of your brain, which develops intuition and an ability to control your mind and actions.

The Moon Center

When you focus your closed eyes downward toward your chin, you are focusing on the Moon Center. This focus is cooling, calming for your emotions, and gives you the insight to see yourself clearly.

The Crown Chakra

When you close your eyes and focus upward toward the top of your head, you are focusing on your Crown Chakra, or the Tenth Gate. When you focus your eyes in this way, it feels as if you are looking through the top of your head. This focus can bring a feeling of elevated spirit and expansion.

One-Tenth Open

When the eyes are indicated to be one-tenth open, allow your eyelids to feel light and relaxed and close your eyes almost all the way, but still allow a bit of light to come into your eyes. This small amount of light will keep your system stimulated and grounded even as you enter into deep meditative states.

Mental Focus—Mantra, Breath, and Visualization

Every element of the universe is manifested to us as light, sound, and energy, and is in a constant state of vibration. Your senses perceive only a fraction of the infinite range of these vibrations. However, you can tune your mind in to the awareness of vibrations with the use of sound and mantra. By vibrating, by chanting in rhythm with your breath and using a particular sound, you expand your sensitivity to include the entire spectrum of vibrations. As you vibrate by thinking, speaking, breathing, and doing, the universe vibrates with you! Kundalini Meditation is based on the premise that your body is a divine instrument and will respond to both the thoughts you have and to the vibrations in the world around you.

Your thoughts can be considered your own inner sounds or vibrations. Meditation can help you form inner vibrations that uplift you, stabilize your identity, and calm your mind and body. There are specific sounds that create positive impressions and elevate your thoughts. These specific sounds link your finite being with the divine vibrations that represent the highest and purest vibrations present within all beings. These sounds are called mantras.

The explanation of how mantras work is scientific. The sounds you vibrate stimulate energetic channels on the roof of your mouth, sending specific signals to your brain. When a mantra is repeated, the signals sent are signals that match divine vibrations. Different mantras are designed to heal specific physical and mental imbalances. Many meditations in this book use mantras. These mantras are an important element in the achievement of the benefits of the meditation.

Creating sound is both a science and an art in which you use your body as an instrument, a vibratory vessel. Before chanting either aloud or silently, follow these steps to add depth, sacredness, and impact to your experience:

1. Take a few relaxed breaths. Bring your attention to your breath and your environment. Listen to the sounds around you. Become sensitive to your space and thoughts—notice your internal and external environments.

2. Bring your awareness to your spine. Visualize your spinal column, and, within that column, a filament pathway in the center. You are visualizing the Central Channel, or *Shushmana*. Now visualize an area in your forehead between your eyebrows and up a bit from the top of your nose. This general area is called the Brow Point. (The Brow Point is referred to in yogic teachings as the great chamber of the pineal gland.) When you create a sound, place it in these areas.

3. When you chant, listen to your own sound with total attention. As you listen, surrender your whole being into the sound you are creating. This will deepen the effects of chanting and prevent your mind from wandering.

Some mantras can be chanted with music; however, it is not recommended to play music during your meditation practice unless a mantra or music is indicated. The meditation itself works on your mind in a specific way for a desired result, and adding music or other

REPETITIVE MEDITATIVE CHANTING

The mind has to be given the medicine of thought. Higher thought is the medicine of the mind that allows it to help itself cure itself. Otherwise the mind is a shattered piece of glass. That is why we do the japa (meditation technique of repetition of a mantra).

—YOGI BHAJAN

If you like to chant and feel uplifted by the practice, choose a mantra that you are drawn to, and repeat it randomly throughout the day, daily during your meditation practice, and in times of challenge. This practice can heal the effects of scars or traumas in your brain and mind, thus healing imbalances in your temperament and personality. When you practice meditations with a mantra, you are planting a seed of divinity in yourself. When that seed takes root and begins to grow, you may start to hear that mantra within you even when you are not meditating. You may wake up in the morning chanting and singing the mantra instead of complaining or thinking that you are too tired to get up. When you have a moment of waiting in line, your mind may return to the mantra instead of becoming frustrated.

After further practice, not only will your mind repeat the mantra, but also you may feel as if the whole universe chants with you. This is the state of *A Jaapa Jaap*. In this state you are identifying with the mantra of truth that you chose. You are linking yourself with the truth, divine energy, and the reality of the meaning and vibration of the mantra. This is a blissful state, a state that can be naturally experienced through regular meditation practice.

If you have had difficulty meditating in the past, try using a mantra as your guide. Choose a mantra and repeat it often. Let it work for you!

external elements may change the intended effect. During quiet breath meditations, you may try listening to a mantra tape softly in the background. Some are suggested at the end of the book. (See page 172.) Mantra music rather than popular music is suggested because of the nature of its vibration—mantra music tends to be less distracting and creates fewer emotional responses than popular music.

In some cases, the mental focus of a meditation may be your breath. The effect of listening to the sound of your breath can be similar to the effect of chanting a mantra. Visualization is also used as another way to focus the mind. These elements of mental focus—breath, mantra, and visualization—are invaluable aids in achieving unbroken concentration during meditation, making your meditation practices highly effective and powerful.

Just like any other skill, concentration improves with practice. You will notice that the meditations in this book include suggested durations of meditation. You are always free to reduce the times of meditations if needed until you learn the skills of particular breath or meditation practice, and slowly increase to the maximum times recommended. While you may choose to reduce the time spent practicing any meditation, it is important not to meditate for *longer* than is indicated for any specific meditation. Certain times are indicated for optimal practice such as 3 minutes, 11 minutes, 22 minutes, 62 minutes, and so on. Yoga masters worked out these time periods based on their specific effects. Here is a list of the basic time segments that you may choose and their effects:

3 minutes—Positively affects the circulation of blood.

11 minutes—Positively affects your nervous system and glandular system.

22 minutes—Balances your Negative, Positive, and Neutral Minds (see page 63).

31 minutes—Triggers the glands, breath, and concentration to affect all the cells and rhythms of the body and deeply affects all layers of your mind.

62 minutes—Brings the positive pattern of the meditation to the brain, which brings the positive effects of the meditation to your nervous system on a deep and long-lasting level.

2½ hours—Some meditations can be practiced for as long as 2½ hours! The practice of this length of meditation can be quite challenging, and the effects can be profound. During a 2½ hour meditation, your subconscious mind will dump its negative impressions and will align with the expansive and uplifting experience of your core spiritual identity.

It is recommended to keep track of time by using a simple programmable digital timer with a soft beep.

Relaxation and Meditation

Once you have begun meditating, you should find yourself feeling more relaxed and at ease. Relaxation, however, is not the same as meditation. While you are meditating, you are using your will to concentrate and to stay focused. During relaxation, you are letting go. When you relax, you are allowing the earth's gravity to hold you, the universe to breathe for you, and letting time and space carry you.

It is common to practice yoga exercises and deep relaxation prior to beginning your meditation session. Exercises like walking, yoga stretching, and yoga postures help your body to relax by releasing minor physical tensions in the body. Walking or yoga practice prior to meditation can also help energize your body by increasing circulation and glandular activity so you can hold focus more efficiently during your meditation session. It is generally recommended to practice deep relaxation again after meditation, to let your mind and body rest deeply. The period of relaxation after you meditate allows the beneficial shifts in mind and body to integrate into your being.

STUDY THE MASTERS OF MEDITATION

The study of the teachings of meditation masters can greatly support your meditation practice. If you have a special teacher, poet, artist, sage, or saint that inspires you, study his or her teachings regularly. When you study the wisdom of the masters, you can embody the strength of that wisdom and you can incorporate the qualities of the masters into your own life. This is a powerful way to augment your meditation practice, and it can bring profound results. Read wisdom teachings regularly before and/or after your meditation practice. For many women, reading inspiring wisdom as taught by meditation masters is itself a powerful meditation.

Relaxation is traditionally practiced by lying on your back, arms by your sides, and palms facing up. This posture allows the body to breathe easily and relax. (You may enjoy covering yourself with a blanket to feel even cozier.) The key to this simple relaxation posture is to be comfortable enough to let your muscles and mind relax. You may also try lying on your belly with your head to one side and your arms in a comfortable position. Relaxing on your belly may feel safer to you if you have experienced sexual traumas or shocks or if you are feeling insecure.

Meditation—mastering the flow and direction of your thoughts—is often the missing key to living a life of grace with a happy and relaxed approach. Relaxation practices that do not include meditation or fail to go deeply into assisting a woman in making healing changes in her thinking often fail to yield lasting results.

The combination of meditation and relaxation brings the depth of rest that women need to clear the many layers of stress that can accumulate physically and mentally. Through practice, your body and mind will learn to recognize the states of tension and relaxation, and you will more easily be able to choose to return to a relaxed state when confronted with inner or outer signals to be tense.

2

Preparing to
Practice

While meditation is certainly an exercise of the mind, it also makes demands of the body. If possible, you should warm up your body before you meditate. A good warm-up can help bridge the gap between daily activity and the stillness of meditation. In order to prepare to meditate, it is suggested to both stretch the body and stimulate circulation so you will have available energy to sustain your meditation practice. In addition to the following exercises and stretches, walking or other aerobic exercise can also be an effective warm-up for meditation.

The sitting postures generally used in meditation may require physical stamina, particularly stamina of the back muscles. If you need to support your back while sitting, try sitting on a yoga cushion, a firm pillow, or a meditation bench. You will know you need support for your back and hips if, when you sit in cross-legged position, your knees are far off the floor and higher than your hips. This means your hips are tight and your back is working too hard to keep you in the position. Sit on a cushion high enough so your knees can relax to hip level, or try meditating in a chair. You can also support your knees and hips by placing pillows or rolled blankets under your knees.

Although your body systems (particularly your nervous system) will be quite active during meditation, your muscles and skeleton should remain still for the most part. Sitting still for long periods can be a challenge for many women. The following yoga exercises and postures can help you to meet this challenge. These yoga postures will help strengthen and release tension from your lower back, stretch and open your hips and legs, and release tension from your upper spine. Practice some or all of these postures anytime prior to or after a meditation session, to help your body prepare for or relax after meditation. If time is an issue for you, you can simply go right into meditation without any physical warm-ups. If these exercises feel strenuous or difficult, use any stretches or exercises that help you release tension from your legs, hips, and back.

SITTING FOR MEDITATION

Take the time you need to create a seated meditation posture that works for you. If you become tired or feel too stiff and need to stretch or lie down, do so. In all of these cases, continue meditating. Your body will become stronger with time. The primary focus of meditation is to work with your mind.

Lower Spinal Flex

Sit in Easy Pose and grasp your ankles with both hands. Locate your navel point and pull the navel point in so your back is elongated. Inhale as you flex your spine forward and lift your chest up, arching your back forward. Concentrate on flexing the lower spine with minimal flex in the upper spine. Exhale as you flex your spine backward and tilt your pelvis back. Keep your head and chin level, while keeping your neck relatively still. Concentrate on the movement of your spine and the rhythm of your breath and mentally chant *Sat* (sounds like *sutt)* as you inhale and *Naam* (sounds like *nahm*) as you exhale. Continue this movement 26–108 times, or for 1–3 minutes. To end, inhale deeply and suspend (hold) your breath for 10–30 seconds. Concentrate your energy at your Brow Point just between your eyes. Then rest for 1 minute as you relax and become still.

Benefits: This exercise helps to stretch and strengthen your lower back. Locating your navel point and applying Neck Lock and Root Lock can help stabilize your spine. Adding the mantra *Sat Naam* on each breath begins the process of meditation by providing a mental focus.

Upper Spinal Flex

Sit in Easy Pose. Grasp your knees with your hands. Pull in your navel point so your back is elongated. Inhale and flex your spine forward, concentrating on bringing the flex into your upper spine. As you flex forward, feel your chest lift up toward your chin and your shoulder blades drop downward and toward each other. Keep your attention on your navel point as you exhale and flex your spine backward, allowing your shoulder blades to stretch apart. Keep your neck relatively still. Continue this flexing motion 26–108 repetitions or for 1–3 minutes.

Benefits: This Upper Spinal Flex will help to stretch both your upper spine and your lower spine.

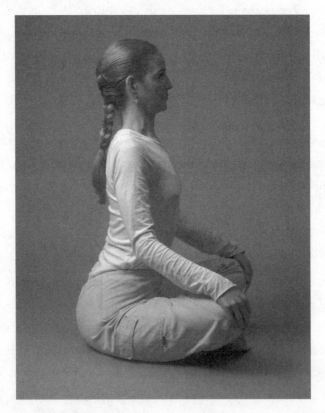

Upper Spinal Flex—Inhalation

LINKING BREATH, MIND, AND BODY

Sat Naam is called a *Bij,* or seed, mantra. In Kundalini Meditation we often mentally chant the *Bij Sat Naam Mantra* in rhythm with the breath. Generally, we chant *Sat* on the inhale and *Naam* on the exhale. *Sat Naam* means truth is my identity. Linking this mantra with the breath focuses your mind and will remind you of your divine identity. This powerful mantra may be used at any time during the day in addition to during meditation and exercise.

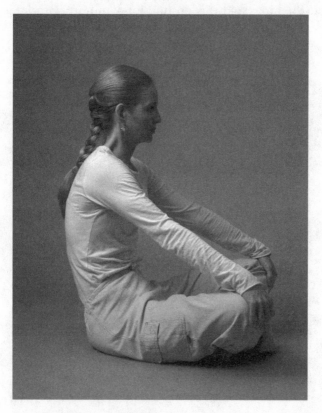

Upper Spinal Flex—Exhalation

Warm-up for Pigeon Pose Lying on Your Back

Lie on your back. Bend your knees with both feet flat on the floor. Lift up your left leg and open your left knee outward, placing your left foot on top of your right thigh, just above your knee. Hold your left shin perpendicular to your right thigh and your left knee pointing out to the left side. Bring your right knee toward your chest, which will press your left shin toward your chest as well. You will feel a stretch in the left hip joint. You can intensify the stretch by clasping your hands around your right leg, just below your knee and gently pulling the right knee toward you. Let your left leg rotate at the hip. Hold this posture for 1 minute with long deep

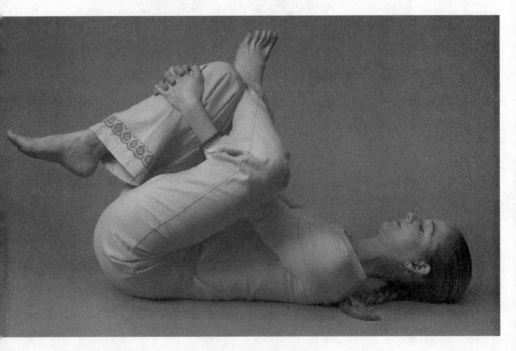

Preparing to Sit for Meditation—Hip Stretch, side view

breathing. Then release the posture. Take a few breaths and switch sides and repeat.

Benefits: This posture will help to stretch your hips and make it easier for you to sit in meditation postures.

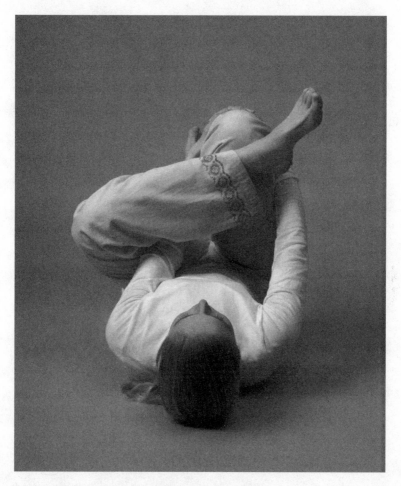

Preparing to Sit for Meditation—Hip Stretch, front view

Pigeon Pose (*Eka Pada Rajakapotasana*)

Sit with the heel of your right foot in front of your pubic bone, with the right foot flexed and your left leg stretched out behind you, with your left kneecap resting on the floor. Place both hands on the floor on each side of your bent right leg.

Variation of Pigeon Pose

If you want a deeper stretch, you can bend forward and lie over your front leg, stretching your arms over your head on the floor. Breathe slowly and deeply. Let go of any tension in your hips. Hold the position for 30 seconds to 1 minute, or as long as is comfortable. Gently come out of the posture by pressing your hands into the floor on each side of your bent left leg, and sit up. Draw your left leg out from under you and relax. Switch sides and repeat.

Benefits: This posture, which can be more challenging than Pigeon Pose Lying on your Back, will help to stretch your hips and make it easier to sit in meditation postures. Choose either one, or both, for an excellent hip stretch.

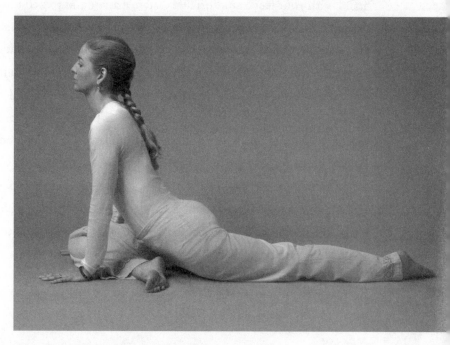

Pigeon Pose (*Eka Pada Rajakapotasana*)

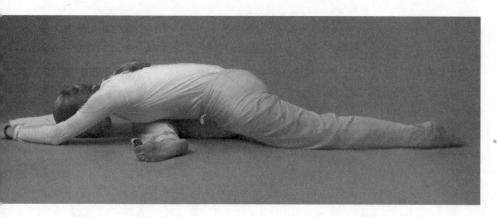

Variation of Pigeon Pose

Heart Opener

Stand with your feet a comfortable distance apart and rooted into the earth, with the crown of your head lifted. This is called Mountain Pose, or *Tadasana*. Apply a light Root Lock, pulling in and up on your navel point. Interlock your hands together behind your lower back, trying to keep your palms together. Keep your shoulder blades lowered on your back and your chest lifted. Inhale and stretch your arms away from your body as your hands lift up and away from your lower back. Be sure not to raise your chin or head as you raise your arms—keep your chin level. Feel your shoulder blades squeeze together. Keeping your arms lifted at a comfortable level, breathe long and deep. Hold this position for up to 1 minute, according to your comfort level. Relax.

Benefits: This posture will help to open and stretch your upper back, bringing relief to tension that you may hold in your upper back.

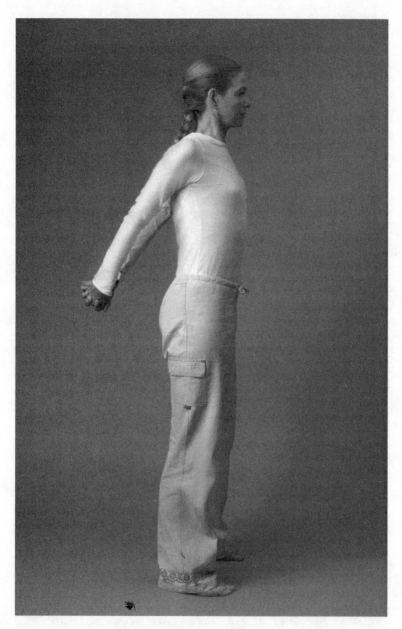

Heart Opener—Standing Shoulder Stretch

Seated Heart Opener

Sit in Easy Pose or a comfortable seated posture. Raise your right
arm straight up and roll your right armpit inward and toward your
head. Bend the right elbow and reach back and down along your
spine with your right palm facing your spine. Bend your left elbow,
rolling your left armpit down and toward your back, and bring your
left arm behind your lower back, with the palm of the left hand fac-

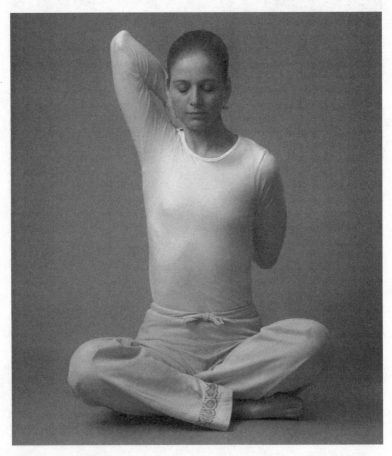

Cowface Pose (*Gomukhasana*) in Easy Pose—Stretching the Upper Body

ing outward. If you can, curl the fingers of the right and left hands and hold the hands together. If your hands cannot reach each other in back, use a yoga strap, towel, or rope between them to complete the connection. Be sure to lift your chest, keep your chin level, and bring your shoulder blades toward each other—as your shoulder blades slide toward each other your elbows open up and away from each other. Be careful not to strain your shoulder joint. Your upper body is in the yoga posture called Cowface Pose, or *Gomukhasana*.

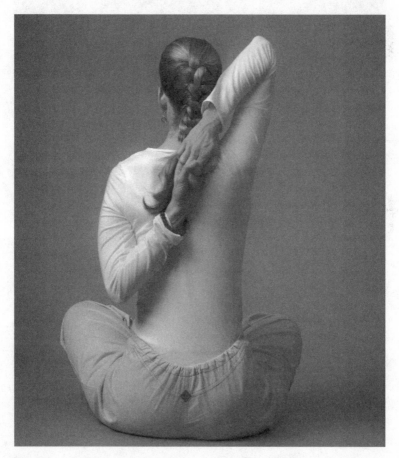

Cowface Pose (*Gomukhasana*) in Easy Pose: view from the back

Hold the posture with long deep breathing for up to 1 minute. Slowly release the posture and relax. Reverse sides and repeat.

Benefits: This posture will help to stretch your upper back, shoulders, and chest.

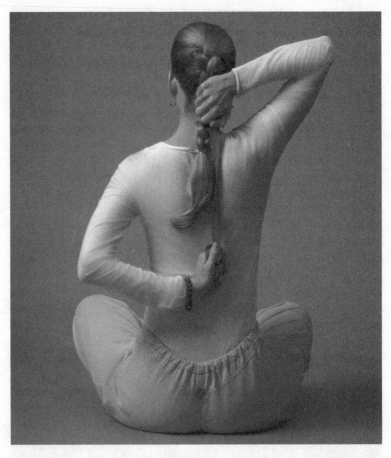

Cowface Pose (*Gomukhasana*) in Easy Pose—Supported Stretch with Yoga Strap

The Swan (*Hansa Kriya*)

Sit in Rock Pose, seated on your heels. Add a blanket or pillow between your heels and buttocks if needed. Place your hands on the floor just beside your knees. Inhale and flex your spine forward, extending your neck to stretch in alignment with your spine. As you exhale, flex your spine backward, opening up your shoulder blades. Still exhaling, dip down, like a swan, bringing your head to the floor. Inhale when your head is at the floor and flex your spine forward again as you come into an upright position. Continue the rhythmic flowing exercise in harmony with your breath 26–108 times. To end, inhale and come sitting up straight into Rock Pose and relax.

Benefits: This posture is especially healing for women. It stretches your entire spine and upper and lower regions of the back. Keeping the breath flowing delivers much-needed energy and massage to your spine and reproductive organs as you stretch. This is an excellent daily practice for women.

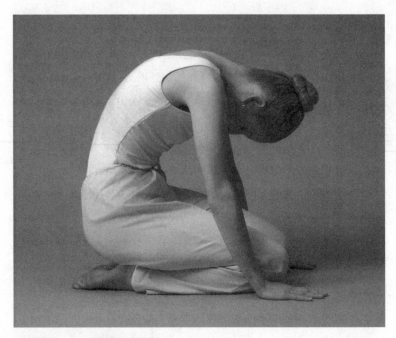

The Swan (*Hansa Kriya*), step one

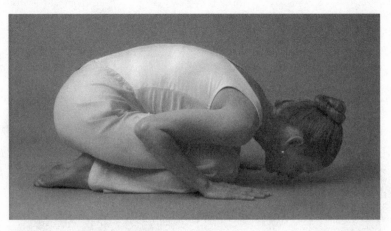

The Swan (*Hansa Kriya*), step two

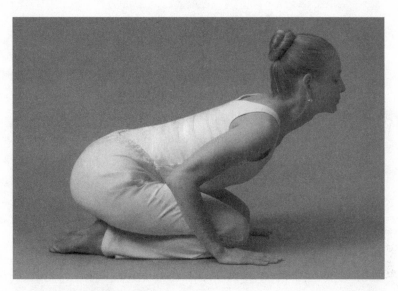

The Swan (*Hansa Kriya*), step three

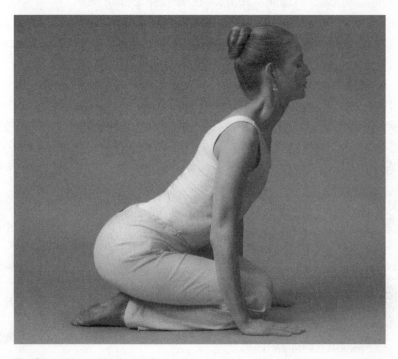

The Swan (*Hansa Kriya*), step four

Life-Nerve Stretch (Head to Knee Pose) (*Paschimottanasana*)

Sit with your spine erect and your legs stretched out in front of you. Keeping your legs close together, root into the ground through your sitting bones and feel your tailbone weighted into the earth. Locate your navel point and pull in and up on the muscles of your lower abdominal area. Lean down from your hips and reach forward with your arms to grasp your toes. Relax your spine and allow your nose to come toward your knees and your elbows to bend and relax down toward the floor. When you stretch down, bend forward from your hip hinge joint, not your waist, and keep your chest open and your heart center lifted. Hold this posture for up to 1 minute with long deep breaths. To end, inhale, suspend your breath briefly, and, pulling your navel point inward to stabilize your lower back, sit up and relax.

If the muscles of your lower and upper back and your hamstrings (the backs of your upper thighs) are tight, you may not be able to reach your toes. If this is the case, sit on a pillow, resting

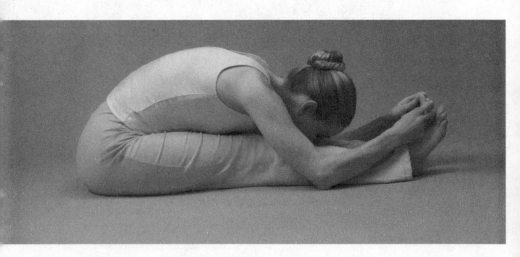

Head to Knee Pose (*Paschimottanasana*), Front Stretch

your hands on your shins or knees as you bend forward from your hips, or use a strap or towel to wrap around your feet. Stretch your hamstrings by flexing your feet and pressing your heels away from you and pressing the backs of your legs into the floor.

Benefits: This yoga pose will help to release stress and stretch your legs and lower back. In this pose you are not only stretching your muscles but also stimulating the large nerves in your legs that connect with your parasympathetic nervous system, which helps you to regain harmony in stressful situations. Practice this posture when you feel stress or to release tension prior to and after meditation.

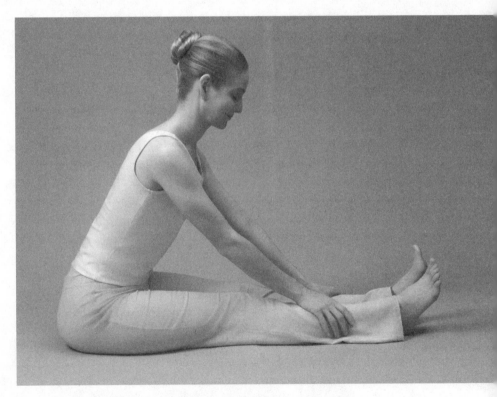

Head to Knee Pose (*Paschimottanasana*), Front Stretch Alternative

Preparing Your Mind for Meditation

In addition to preparing the body for meditation, it is also important to prepare the mind. Remembering your primary intention—the goal of your meditation practice—before you begin meditating can be helpful to your practice. Before you meditate, give yourself permission to let go of any fears or concerns about your schedule, your responsibilities, or whatever else might be on your mind. Remind yourself that the purpose of your meditation practice is to provide a healing space for yourself. Trust that for the length of time of your meditation you can relax all of your concerns and that your world will remain intact. Remember that your responsibilities will still be there when you finish meditating, and you'll be more able to fulfill them!

The Body-Mind Experience of Meditation

Besides becoming aware of your thoughts and the flow of your mental activity during meditation, you will most likely feel many physical sensations as you practice. These sensations can be pleasurable and include both a gradual or sudden relaxation of your muscles and/or chronic tension, pleasurable movements of energy in your body, and a tingling or warm sensation; however, you may also experience stiffness in your hips, legs falling asleep, or back discomfort at times. Fortunately, there are ways to handle both the physical discomforts that may occur during meditation and any distracting thoughts that come to your mind.

Some physical discomforts can be a result of mental activity. If your mind is very jumpy and resists your efforts at sitting still, your mind may then send messages to your body to shift positions. Each time you feel that you need to shift positions or stretch, ask yourself this question: "Is this movement needed by my physical body or is this just my mind transferring its jumpy nature to my body?" Part of the process of meditation is learning this distinction. If you sense that your mind is trying to trick you to prevent you from becoming still, don't make the physical adjustment. Often your mind will transfer the desire to move to another part of the body, or it will let go of the thought altogether.

However, if you feel a real need to stretch or move your body during your meditation session, take a break and relax. To avoid losing concentration, you may choose to continue your mantra and breathing during your stretching break.

Keep up! As with any physical practice, your ability to sit and meditate will improve as you practice. Meditation is an ongoing process. Although meditation can bring immediate results, the deeper benefits come from practice over a period of time.

Thoughts During Meditation

When you begin to meditate and try to focus your mind on a breathing technique, mantra, or any other focal point, your mind will begin to naturally generate unrelated thoughts. As you meditate, thoughts and memories that were previously hidden from you—in your subconscious mind—may begin to come into your conscious mind. This is a positive sign—once your thoughts move from your subconscious mind into your conscious mind you will be able to process them.

CONCENTRATION TIPS

One of the biggest challenges in meditation is to maintain your concentration. Here are a few ways to help you hold your concentration during a meditation session.

- If your mind is tired, you may feel physically tired, and vice versa. When you feel tired, think thoughts that will uplift and inspire you. For example: "If I keep up with this, I will feel the benefits of meditation and be more focused in my life." Then return your focus to the particular meditation technique you are practicing.
- If your mind is overexcited, think thoughts that will calm you down, thoughts that trigger the expansive and vast qualities of the mind. For example: "I am meditating to create peace in my heart, peace on earth, peace in this universe."
- Try not to overconcentrate. If you notice your face in a frown or your body tensing up during meditation, you may be overconcentrating. Take a moment to relax your mind and body as you hold the posture steady. There is an art to balancing the concentration and relaxation involved in meditation. Seek this balance as you practice.
- If concentration is difficult for you, try meditating for shorter periods of time. Start with as little as three minutes and build up from there. Success in meditation practice will come if you start where you are, have realistic expectations, and have patience with the process.

Sometimes your thoughts during meditation can be pleasant and generate happy and peaceful sensations, but sometimes the thoughts may generate unpleasant sensations. The thoughts that trigger unpleasant sensations may be memories of the past or fears of the future. Do not try to avoid having these types of thoughts. These very thoughts are coming up so you can dump them, so you can become free from the memories that bind you to the past and keep you from seeing the world as it is. If you notice unpleasant thoughts or memories during your meditation session, allow them to come and go without identifying with them or adding any additional distress to their appearance. Simply notice your thoughts as they arise and bring your attention repeatedly and patiently back to the meditation technique. Trust the process—the meditation itself will naturally cleanse your subconscious mind and will heal negative thinking patterns and past psychic wounds.

Do not be surprised by how potent meditation can be in revealing the inner workings of your mind and thoughts. If you find that your meditations repeatedly bring up disturbing memories, seek support from a therapist or teacher to help you move through the self-healing process. As you embrace, accept, and forgive yourself for the past and start to understand and release your fears, you are on the path to self-healing. Your mind will begin to be more present instead of dwelling in the past or projecting into the future.

Don't react to your thoughts by creating a "thought train." A thought train occurs when you give your attention to one thought and it leads to another and another. One original thought may lead to an entire mental scenario, which can then stimulate desires and emotions. Instead of becoming enmeshed in a thought train, simply notice your thoughts. Notice also that you have lost concentration on the focal point of the meditation. When you bring your mind back to the focal point, you will be amazed to see that a thought train, which may have caused a strong reaction with spin-off desires and emotions, completely vanishes without a trace in seconds! Each meditation session includes a steady stream of this type of interaction with your mind. When you meditate, you are scientifically training your mind to stay steady instead of moving chaotically about as a result of your thoughts.

TOTAL RELAXATION

Meditation can help relieve the deeper levels of accumulated stress. Women have a natural capacity for operating on many levels simultaneously. This ability is unique to women and can be both an advantage and disadvantage. On the plus side, this natural capacity allows a woman to simultaneously fulfill her roles as mother, wife, businessperson, and so on. Some even say that women have an advantage in business and politics as a result of this capacity. Yogi Bhajan teaches that women operate on six levels at once, while men operate on only one level. The challenge of this expanded capacity is that in order to maintain all six levels, women need to learn to relax all six levels. Meditation accesses and relaxes all the levels of a woman's being and gives a woman an opportunity to clear her mind. Total relaxation is a result of mental relaxation, physical relaxation, and the realization that you have a strong core identity that includes self-respect.

Your First Meditation Session

Here is the basic sequence of a meditation session:

1. Tune In and Create a Sacred Space. When you practice Kundalini Yoga and Meditation as taught by Yogi Bhajan, you "tune in" with a mantra before you begin your practice. The recitation of the mantra creates a sacred space for your practices and links you with the meditation masters (the Golden Link) who have come before you.

    To tune in, sit in a relaxed meditative posture with your hands in Prayer Pose, most commonly called *Atmanjali Mudra,* both hands in front of your chest with your palms together. Close your eyes and take a few deep breaths. Then repeat the following mantra aloud, as indicated below. Repeat the mantra 3 times or more, until you feel ready to begin your practice.

Ong Namo Guru Dev Namo
Ong – ng namo
gu – roo (on the *r,* hit your tongue on the roof of your mouth)
dayv namo

Which means:

I acknowledge the One Creative Consciousness.
I acknowledge the Subtle and Divine Wisdom Within.

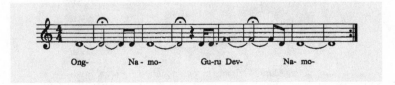

Musical Notation for *Ong Namo Guru Dev Namo*

2. Choose and practice any warm-up yoga postures or breathing techniques to help you prepare for meditation.

3. Settle into a comfortable seated meditation posture.

4. Meditate. Follow the directions of your chosen meditation, including times. To begin your practice, you may choose a meditation from the three meditations included in this section or any other meditation from this book that inspires you.

5. End the meditation as indicated.

6. Relax. Take some time to stretch and relax on your back after meditation.

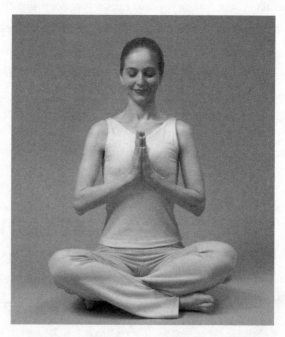

Atmanjali Mudra—Tuning In for Meditation in Prayer Pose

7. Sit up and take a moment to project an intention or affirmation for peace and healing for yourself, someone you know, and/or the world.

The meditations that follow are good meditations for beginners. Practice one or more of these simple meditations every day or as frequently as you are able. These meditations are great to return to when you need centering and rejuvenation.

 ## Breath Awareness Meditative Exercise

By practicing this breath meditation, you will become aware of your baseline of energy—in Sanskrit called *prana*. If you can sense the ups and downs of your own energy flow, you can develop the ability to balance your energy, conserve it, and direct it as needed in your life.

Sit with a straight spine in a relaxed meditative pose. Let your hands rest over the knees in *Gyan Mudra* (touching the tip of your index finger to the tip of your thumb and resting your wrists on your knees), or keep them in Prayer Pose (palms together in front of your chest) at the center of the chest. Let your body feel in perfect balance. You can sit in this posture without effort. Let your entire attention gather on the breath. Sense the breath as a quality of motion. How does it move in the different parts of your body as you breathe in a steady and meditative rhythm? Do you feel tired and excited or balanced and relaxed? How does your experience change as you continue to meditate?

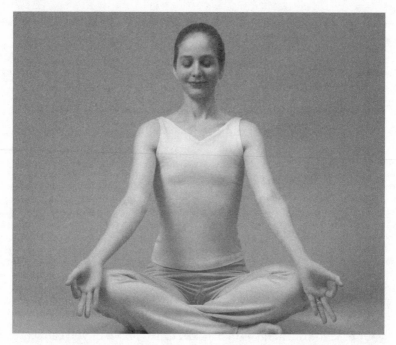

Easy Pose utilizing *Gyan Mudra*—Breath Awareness Meditative Exercise

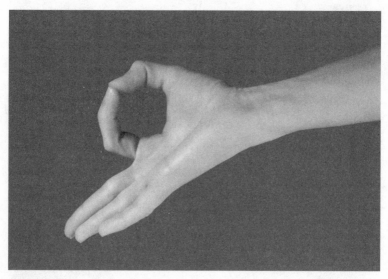

Gyan Mudra

Bring your attention through the one-inch-square area above the root of the nose where the eyebrows meet—the Brow Point. Then focus the attention through the brow onto the navel point.

Feel the motion and life energy of your breath. Visualize your body as luminous. As you inhale, the light increases in brightness, extent, and penetration. Let that breath and light merge with the entire cosmos. Feel that you are a part of that vastness. The breath is a wave on a much greater ocean of energy of which you are a part. Continue this visualization for 3–62 minutes.

 ## Meditation for Relaxing Body and Mind

If you have thoughts during the meditation, keep bringing your focus back to the mantra and let the mantra work to cut through the chaos of your mind.

Sit in a meditation posture with your spine straight. Place your hands in *Gyan Mudra*. Begin slow Long Deep Yogic Breathing (as described on page 15). With each inhalation, mentally chant the mantra *Sat*. With each exhalation, mentally chant the mantra *Naam*. Continue for 3–11 minutes, allowing your breath to become deep and slow and conscious.

Calming the Nervous System— Alternative Nostril Breathing Meditation (*Nadi-Sodhana*)

The energy of the nervous system is directly proportional to one's breathing. Ancient yogic texts explain that your right (sun) nostril controls your energy level; your left (lunar) nostril controls your emotions. Consequently, breathing long and deep through the right nostril will give you added energy, while breathing through the left nostril will bring you calmness even in the midst of strong emotions like anger, nervousness, joy, and sadness. This particular technique is a simple but effective way to quickly restore your balance when you feel off-center and yet must still function in the world. For instance, a teenage girl may feel emotional or nervous and still need to go to school, take tests, and be in social environments. This technique can help her calm herself so she can function more effectively and feel happier.

Sit in a meditative posture with your spine straight. Make a U shape with the thumb and pinky finger of your right hand. Use your thumb to close off your right nostril and your pinky finger to close off your left nostril while practicing the following breath sequence.

Close your left nostril and inhale deeply through your right nostril. At the completion of your inhale close your right nostril and exhale through your left nostril. Inhale again, this time through your left nostril. Then close your left nostril and exhale through your right one. Continue this alternating breathing pattern for 3–5 minutes. Make an effort to fully inhale and completely exhale your breath. To end the meditation, inhale deeply, hold the breath a few seconds, then lower your hand, and exhale. Relax and enjoy a feeling of well-being!

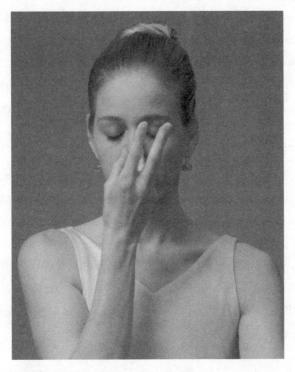

Alternate Nostril Breathing Meditation—*Nadi-Sodhana:* calming the nervous system

4/4 Breath for Energy and Focus

Segmented breathing works quickly to relax you by slowing your breath rate and to energize you by intensifying your focus and awareness. This type of breathing also safely exercises your abdominal muscles. The muscles move slightly with each segment, stretching with the inhalation and moving toward your spine with the exhalation. Many women find that segmented breathing revitalizes their energy and relieves stressful thoughts.

Sitting in Easy Pose, take a few long, deep breaths. Then begin inhaling in 4 short segments and exhaling in 4 segments. Breathe through your nose and go at a pace that is comfortable; you should not feel strained or out of breath. Continue for 1–3 minutes, or up to 11 minutes, and then relax. You can try other breath ratios, such as inhaling 8 segments, then exhaling 8 segments, and so on. To deepen the experience, link your breath with a mental recitation of the mantra *Saa Taa Naa Maa.*

A MANTRA FOR TRANSITIONS

Saa Taa Naa Maa is called the *Panj Shabad,* which means the five sounds of life: *S, T, N, M,* and *aa.* These basic syllables are the primal sounds of the mantra *Sat Naam,* the seed mantra of Truth. Each sound creates a unique vibration in your body and mind. These vibrations have the effect of stimulating a particular state of mind, according to their meanings:

Saa—infinity, cosmos, beginning, and birth

Taa—life, existence

Naa—death, totality, and transition

Maa—rebirth and renewal

QUESTIONS FOR REFLECTION

After you meditate ask yourself:

- Were you able to find and sustain a comfortable seated posture?

- Were you able to complete the meditation?

- What feelings, thoughts, or emotions did you experience during your meditation session?

- Did you notice a shift in your mental state after the meditation session?

3

The Nature of
Your Mind

T ry this experiment. Sit down, still your body, and focus once again on your breath. After 3 minutes, evaluate your experience. Here are a few questions for reflection:

1. Did you have thoughts?

2. Did you have feelings about those thoughts?

3. Did you act on all of your thought impulses?

Did you have any thoughts? Of course you did! It is natural for your mind to create thoughts. These thoughts can be random, organized, linear, nonlinear, happy, sad, empowering, or disempowering. Your thoughts may be a combination of many different types that generate many different feelings and emotions. The yogis say that your mind generates a thousand thoughts per blink of your eye! Take a moment to write down a few of the thoughts you had during the exercise. Would you say that all of these thoughts truly represent who you really are? Were all of your thoughts worthy of being acted upon? Most people would answer with a resounding no!

It is important to realize that you do not need to identify with your thoughts. Many people describe their first experience of silent meditation—simply becoming aware of their own thinking—to be enlightening. Although most women would like their minds to be more peaceful, many of us are not aware that the very thoughts we are habitually generating can be causing discomfort. Without training in meditation, people generally assume that it is what is happening *outside oneself* that causes discomfort. When you experience and accept that it may be *your own thinking* that is causing your pain, your healing journey through meditation can begin.

The yogis believe that there is an intrinsic truth to our nature that is beyond thought. This core identity is timeless, beautiful, and blissful. Finding and holding your core identity, then, is simply reconnecting to, or remembering, the higher part of you that is already present. The reason why many women do not experience this core identity is because the mind has developed the habit of concentrating on the chaos and distractions of the world and the senses. Through the practice of meditation you can learn to let go of these limiting attention patterns and focus instead on the various aspects of your core identity. Guru Nanak, an enlightened saint and yogi once said, very simply, "If you master your mind, you master the world."

Let's talk about how your mind works so you can gain the self-knowledge to meditate and experience a core identity of truth and bliss.

The Negative, Positive, and Neutral Aspects of Your Mind

Yogi Bhajan, Master of Kundalini Yoga, has identified the three most basic aspects of the human mind. These aspects are called the Negative, or Protective Mind, the Positive, or Projective Mind, and the Neutral, or Meditative Mind. Understanding how these three minds function is the key to unlocking the secrets of our complex thinking process.

The Negative Mind

The negative mind is a protector developed to preserve your life. It can give you a powerful self-understanding and detailed critiques of your actions. It can tell you what is wrong, what might be harmful, and locate problems to be solved.

—YOGI BHAJAN

Your Negative Mind is the first part of your mind to engage when you confront any situation. The Negative Mind engages first in order to assess the situation and protect you from danger. The Negative Mind is both sensitive and subtle, like a vigilant guard that checks out your environment and reports any perceived dangers to your conscious mind. Women have a strong protective mind, partially because we hold the future generations in our wombs. This strong natural instinct for self-preservation combined with an expanded sensitivity and alertness to the environment is intended to protect and secure the future generations that women are responsible for.

The Positive Mind

If the Negative Mind serves as a protector, then the Positive Mind serves as your representative. The Positive Mind evaluates any situation to determine how you can use the situation for furthering your goals and interests. Then it uses the information it gathers to compare the present to the past and possible futures. This function of the Positive Mind can balance the Negative Mind by challenging or supporting the warnings of the Negative Mind, leading you to reevaluate the situation.

The Negative and Positive Minds in Action

The thoughts that the Positive and Negative Minds create are often in conflict with each other or are polarities of each other, as neither in themselves can see the whole picture. They both serve an important purpose but are limited in their ability to work together to come to a balanced conclusion. Even if you are not aware of the interplay between the Negative and Positive Minds, you are often aware of the confusion that is created by this interplay when you're having difficulty making decisions.

Sometimes when you try to work out an important issue or make an important decision, you think it through and still find yourself confused or find yourself wavering between different conclusions. In order to clearly navigate through the activity of the Negative and Positive Minds and their spin, you must be able to listen to yourself through your own Neutral, or Meditative Mind.

The Positive Mind and the Negative Mind are constantly engaged with your environment, processing every thought and interpreting and assessing each experience. Their interactions create new thoughts that are a continuous commentary on the perceived situation. Together they are like political commentators creating political spin. If you try to listen to the Positive and Negative Minds simultaneously, you can forget the original issue, get lost in the commentary, and be tempted to react with emotion and passion to the extremes of the commentary.

If you don't deal with your thoughts through the meditative aspect of your mind, you will inevitably spin off into thoughts of the past and projections into the future. You will not be living in the present. You may lose the thread of a conversation, for example, and begin relating to a person through your past, or you may misinterpret the intention of the other person. The spinning and cloaking qualities of the Positive and Negative Minds can bring a wavering or confused quality to your thinking.

The Neutral Mind

First you have to walk out into the Neutral/Meditative Mind, which must tell you what is right and what is wrong, and that is where the juice of life is. That's where happiness is. That's where the future is. —YOGI BHAJAN

Your Neutral, or Meditative, Mind is the aspect of your mind that has the capacity to see the big picture. The Meditative Mind can see how the Negative and Positive Minds are working together. Living in your Meditative Mind is like residing on the peak of a mountain. From this mountain peak you can see the workings of both the Negative (Protective) and the Positive (Projective) Minds as they engage each situation. You can clearly see the reality of the world you are living in. You can assess the information gathered from the Negative and Positive Minds and make clear decisions. The Meditative Mind is your intuition; it is your meditative perspective, your divine vision. The practice of meditation gives you the experience of the clarity and peace of your Meditative Mind.

Meditation will teach you how to perceive the thoughts created by the Positive and Negative Minds through the Neutral Mind. Meditation does this by creating a Still Point, a moment when the Meditative Mind is activated, as mentioned in the first chapter. During moments like this the Protective and Projective Minds don't have such a strong pull on your thinking. Through this Still Point, you experience the Meditative Mind. Even as you perceive the activity of your mind, you are no longer entangled with your thoughts. One purpose of meditation is to directly experience the clarity and peace of the Meditative Mind, and to be free from the confusion of spiraling thoughts and their corresponding emotions and feelings.

Guided Visualization to Help You Understand Your Three Minds Inspired by the Teachings of Yogi Bhajan

Try the following meditation exercise to understand the nature of the Negative, Positive, and Meditative aspects of your mind. With practice, you can learn to recognize the qualities of each aspect of your mind. This can lead to better decision making and deeper self-knowledge.

Sit in a relaxed seated posture. Place the hands, palms up, in front of the chest at the level of the heart center. Put the right hand on top of the left hand; fingers of the two hands are at cross angles. Touch the tips of the thumbs together. Elbows are relaxed along the sides. Eyes are closed or one-tenth open.

With a slow breath put your mind through the following three stages of deep self-entrancement and focus. As you breathe slowly, concentrate on each facet of your mind as explained below.

Negative Mind: Let all thoughts come across the inner screen of your mind. Hear all the inner voices. Whatever thought comes, immediately negate it. If the mind says, "I'm a woman," project "I am not a woman." If the mind projects "I'm big," then negate the thought by thinking "I'm not big." If it is a picture that shows "I'm big," imagine that it fades away, or explodes, or changes to something that shows you smaller. Every particular thought is negated, detached from, and let go. In this meditation the habit of the mind to select the same repetitive thoughts is countered by the use of the Negative Mind. Continue for 1–11 minutes.

Positive Mind: Switch to questions that engage the Positive, Projective Mind. Acknowledge your relationship to the world. Ask questions like "How can I use or learn from this experience to express my soul, my core, and my awakened awareness?" "What can I do now to extend myself to the greater life of which I am a part?" Let your mind be creative, exploratory, and free. Connect each thought and feeling to a positive use or learning. Continue for 1–11 minutes.

Neutral Mind: Now switch to statements that affirm and confirm your existence, whole and complete, autonomous and joyful. Immerse your mind in the thought of your own Infinity. Examples are: *I* AM, I *AM;* I am bountiful, I am blissful, I am beautiful. During this meditation you may wish to create an image or metaphor for this infinite connection and dwelling in your essence. Examples of these images or metaphors may be a special environment; an image of a vast ocean of energy and light that you immerse yourself in; a tree that extends its roots deep into the Earth as it extends into the heavens with many fruits or flowers. Let the image be natural to you, but let it capture this feeling of completion, bliss, autonomy, and trust in your higher Self. Continue for 3–31 minutes.

QUESTIONS FOR REFLECTION

- Which facet of the mind was easiest for you to experience? Which facet was the most challenging for you to experience?

- Is there a facet of your mind that is overactive? In other words, do you dwell too much in the Negative Mind or the Positive Mind?

- How did it feel to live from the Meditative Mind? How often do you live from the meditative aspect of your mind?

4

Building a
True Identity

*Woman is the center of Infinity. She is the only reality
the Earth knows. She's the only reality the heaven blesses.*

—YOGI BHAJAN

According to yogic philosophy, a woman's nature
compares to the moon. The moon is reflective,
cool, calm, and shining. When the heat of the
day comes to a cooling, expansion begins. Without the moon,
nothing will expand and grow.

A woman is a beacon of light to show the way. The woman
nurtures and shows the way by sharing her inspiration and her light
in times of darkness. A woman's true nature is like that of a flow-

ing river. She is a constant flow of spiritual energy inspiring the growth of everything she touches.

Just as a woman holds her child in the womb, so does she hold her entire family and the family of humanity in her aura, which can be huge and strong. She is naturally highly sensitive to even the slightest shifts in her environment as she creates a cozy home for all.

A woman is naturally intuitive, and said to possess a power of psyche sixteen times that of a man! If this is so, why do so many women feel powerless, angry, or unfulfilled? Why are women oppressed, exploited, tortured, and abused? Why do so many women, especially young women, who know their truth and have goodness in their hearts, have such difficulty claiming their power and living happily?

Yogi Bhajan lectured for years on this problem. He taught us how we can assist in the empowerment of women and showed us how women can find happiness amid the difficulties inherent in our modern culture. The solution he presented is two-fold. The first part is for the world to understand the basic identity of women and respect it. If women are not respected, our culture will fall short of providing us inner peace and universal love, and all of our wonderful technological achievements will fail to heal us. The position of women must be elevated in order for us to move into an age of elevated consciousness. The second part of the solution is for women to understand and embrace their own identity. Yogi Bhajan teaches that all a woman needs to do is to *identify herself as a woman* and she will feel the empowerment of that identity. By this, Yogi Bhajan means that women should fight the temptation to be defined by disempowering trends and outside influences and, instead, choose an identity that is timeless, uplifting, and real. The feminine psyche has to be strong enough to hold this identity through the challenges of her environment and the pervasive trends of the day. Regular meditation is the practice that develops this core strength.

Let's look at some of the reasons why women may find it difficult to embrace their true identity.

Our "Hiding Nature"

It is common for women in our culture to hide their true selves. Many women find it easier to follow the crowd in order to fit in and find acceptance. Many women also feel safer when hidden. There are theories that consider this hiding nature is due, in part, to the fact that women's sexual organs are hidden within her, not external. The female body is designed to protect and contain children developing in the womb, and this basic biological fact may have greater implications in the development of her psyche.

A woman's tendency toward a hiding nature has both positive and negative manifestations. One negative manifestation of this natural tendency is that women can go through life without expressing their true selves into the world. The positive manifestation of women's hiding nature is a woman's ability to protect her body, her identity, and the power of her being.

Living with a spiritual identity as a woman presents a challenge because it requires a woman to assert her inner truth despite this natural hiding tendency. Without a strong spiritual identity, it is inevitable that one's identity and self-esteem will change along with circumstances and outside pressures. Let's call this the *shaky identity syndrome*. When a woman is living with a shaky identity, she is constantly looking outside herself for validation, she may automatically follow disempowering societal trends, and she may compromise her values for attention, status, or financial gain. With a shaky identity, a woman also may enter into unhealthy relationships in order to fill the emptiness that comes when she does not realize and affirm her true identity as a woman. Living and holding your true identity, then, is as much a matter of what you do as what you don't do. *Keeping your core identity intact through meditation and right action is the way to a positive self-image for women of all ages. It is the key to happiness and spiritual growth.*

The moment a woman finds the power to be her true self, she radiates her infinite nature and she becomes spiritually invincible. The moment a woman identifies herself as a true woman, she is called upon to become great. She is called upon to become fearless. By identifying with the universal concept of woman, she identifies with something beyond her personality, beyond smallness and insecurity. Her actions start to represent something more than just herself—something great, real, and uplifting.

Once you identify yourself, you can represent yourself accurately, and you will accurately represent your skills, your talents, and your potential. You will become bright and self-confident. Although living with a strong identity may be challenging at times, this type of living brings fulfillment in the knowledge that you did not sell yourself short or sell yourself out.

How Meditation Helps You Develop Your True Identity

Creating a strong identity is a matter of choice. Nobody is born a winner, and nobody is born a loser—we are all born choosers. Your mind is vast enough and strong enough to hold any identity you choose. The question is: What are you choosing as your identity? What is your destination in your life, what are you working toward? Do you have the strength and the tools you need to achieve your goals? Have you identified yourself in such a way that you remain inspired to fulfill that identity? This is where meditation comes in.

A meditation practice can help you develop self-confidence and self-knowledge through stabilizing the mind—eliminating the habitual thought patterns that create and fuel a shaky identity. One purpose of meditation, then, is to bring an unshakable stability to your chosen identity. As a result of developing this strength, no outside forces will be able to shake you from the strength of your convictions. In the following chapters, we will examine how your thoughts create your identity and reality. The meditations, relaxation techniques, and exercises in this book are designed to help you on this healing journey.

A WOMAN'S OATH

Put your right hand on your heart and say, "I, the woman born into this body and in this Grace, take an oath of honor. Today and every day shall be noble for me, so help me God." Recite this oath every day as soon as you wake up, and before you go to sleep at night.

VISUALIZE THE TRUE YOU

Sit quietly and comfortably. Focus on the natural process of your breathing. As you feel your breath, visualize yourself as an instrument of Divine energy. Feel Divine energy and music flowing through you. Each breath you take is a musical note that creates a melody. That melody is your body. Your body becomes an expression of the music of your breathing. This exercise helps stimulate your creativity and helps you drop physical tension and a disempowering body image. Try this meditation for 11 minutes and see what happens. Draw the picture you see or journal the story of your experience.

As you develop your meditation practice and begin to feel increasingly secure in your spiritual identity, you will notice changes in your life. You'll move closer to a higher state of stability and self-satisfaction. Whether you describe these changes in spiritual or psychological terms, living in these higher states of mind is deeply empowering. The following descriptions can help you recognize the changes you are likely to experience as you practice meditation and begin to claim your true identity.

The Royal Woman

When a woman rejects society's classifications and identifies herself from within, she develops a strong inner core of values and truth and makes peace with her past. She begins to live more freely. Her attitude is like the attitude of a princess. As she becomes independent of the challenges of the world and the disappointments of the past, an inner royalty manifests itself as outer graciousness and knowledge. At this stage, a woman finds it easier to handle the outer challenges and stresses of life, be they those of a mother, a CEO, or a student. Her mind wavers less and she finds it easier to express herself. Her actions begin to be driven by self-esteem instead of insecurity.

The Radiant Woman

The next stage of the journey appears when a woman embodies the natural feminine aspect of containment. At this stage, a woman's presence becomes so strong that she does not have to say a lot to get attention. Her presence radiates her wisdom in a practical way. Her projection is one of self-confidence, and it creates a pathway for everything to fall in place around her.

The Self-Disciplined Woman

Self-discipline characterizes the third stage of development. This woman's presence inspires others to find their own inner strength. Her sight, touch, existence, talk, imagination, and relationships are an inspiration toward elevation. In this stage, it becomes easy for a woman to hold true to her inner values in all situations.

The Yogini

The Yogini lives in a state in which the pair of opposites do not affect her. In this final stage, the Yogini sees both good and bad simply as polarities in the play of life. She lives in a river of Grace and can flow through challenges and remain calm. Under all situations she radiates forgiveness, blessing, compassion, kindness, and smiles.

I hope these descriptions of some of the stages on the path of self-healing inspire you to begin your meditation practice with commitment, patience, forgiveness, and a willingness to discover, uncover, and live your inner truth. Try not to get discouraged if you slip back into old habits of low self-esteem or negative thought patterns. Setbacks are a natural part of breaking old habits and creating a new identity.

Keep up! The journey of self-healing through meditation can bring these transformations to you.

 A Visualization to Start the Journey

The following meditative visualization, inspired by Yogi Bhajan, is designed to help you feel your royal identity and build self-esteem. You can read it and visualize as you read or record your voice and close your eyes and meditate as you listen.

Sit comfortably and relax your breath. Visualize yourself on a throne. Decorate the throne beautifully, royally, with precious jewels, flowers, or whatever represents prosperity and royalty to you. See yourself dressed as a Queen, a Royal Highness. Hypnotize yourself with complete belief and confidence. See yourself as the Imperial Majesty in your Court. Meditate on this vision of yourself as royal and relaxed.

Benefits: This visualization can help you reclaim the original feminine identity that is your birthright.

5

Science and the Meditative Mind

magine yourself feeling relaxed a good deal of the time. Imagine feeling secure in your identity as a spiritual woman, regardless of outer circumstances. Imagine yourself having the tools to tap into an unlimited source of energy, enthusiasm, and creativity, renewed each day in as little as 20 minutes.

If you find yourself feeling negative about yourself and your world, meditate and feel the joy that is always available to you, despite external circumstances and inner trials! If you are exhausted, mentally and physically, from the demands of work and family, meditate and draw new strength to cope. If you are feeling well, meditate to deepen your well-being and gather strength for the future. If you seek to understand the deeper realities of your spirit and your place in the grand design of life, meditate and discover the priceless treasures within you! All of this, and more, can be yours if you develop your personal meditation practice. I have seen hundreds of women achieve these goals in my fifteen years' teaching Kundalini meditation. The changes I have witnessed have given me an unshakable faith in the potential of the feminine spirit to heal, grow, and expand. Evidence of meditation's benefits abounds in the lives of men and women everywhere, and I trust that you, too, have experienced its tremendous power. For millennia, people who practiced meditation have reported its positive effects on their bodies and minds. A natural question then arises—How does the practice of meditation have these far-ranging effects?

Starting in the 1930s, scientists have been studying the effects of meditation in the laboratory, trying to pinpoint the psychophysical mechanisms that account for the positive changes which occur during meditation practice. As of this writing, there have been literally hundreds of studies that have proved the positive effects of meditation.

Meditation, Stress, and the "Relaxation Response"

In the medical community it is thought that stress accounts for up to two-thirds of all visits to the doctor's office. It is well documented that high levels of long-term stress are a contributing factor to many of the major illnesses suffered in the modern world, from heart disease, diabetes, hypertension, and cardiovascular disease to depression, anxiety, and insomnia.

One way that science has defined stress is as a state of arousal, often brought on by a feeling of being threatened or overchallenged. In this aroused psychophysical state, the sympathetic nervous system is highly charged, resulting in the release of the chemicals adrenaline and cortisol. A host of other changes in the autonomic nervous system are brought about as well, all of which prepare you to deal with the perceived threat (the so-called fight or-flight syndrome). It is this arousal of the body systems, sustained for prolonged periods of time, that is thought to account for the contribution of stress to many illnesses and imbalances.

In the 1970s, researcher Herbert Benson discovered a natural human state of mind and body that he called the "relaxation response." The relaxation response, which has successfully been duplicated by researchers around the globe, is characterized by the *exact opposite* response in the body, and this response can be achieved through meditation. After only twenty minutes daily of practicing meditation with a mantra, sympathetic nervous system activity was reduced, parasympathetic activity (responsible for creating and sustaining the states of relaxation) was increased, heart rate and oxygen consumption were lowered, and the meditator reported a heightened sense of well-being and alertness. It was also demonstrated that subjects who were the most stressed obtained the greatest benefits from their meditation sessions.

These proven scientific differences between the stress response and the relaxation response are the best evidence of meditation's wide-ranging effects. In addition, it has been shown that the longer one continues practicing meditation regularly, the greater the positive benefits.

Meditation and Heart Rate

When we break the relaxation response into just two of its components, we see further the physical benefits of meditation. Numerous studies attest to the reduction of the average heart rate. In fact, one study found that people who meditate regularly with a mantra for four or more years had an average heart rate drop of 9 percent.

This finding was later reported by researchers who in 1982 divided sixty subjects into six groups. Each group was taught a different technique designed to elicit a state of relaxation. The results indicated that the group taught meditation with a mantra lowered their heart rate an average of seven beats per minute, as compared with other techniques of which the best (biofeedback) lowered the heart rate only 3 beats per minute. As the stressful state of "fight or flight" normally raises the heart rate, a lowered rate is an indication of a more relaxed, tranquil state of body and mind.

Meditation and Hypertension

But meditation affects more than just the heart rate. The scientific studies that have been done to observe the effect of meditation on people with hypertension have been exciting and surprising, and their discoveries have great promise in the treatment of mild and moderate high blood pressure. The findings have shown systolic reductions of up to 25 mmHg or more that have been replicated to date in more than nineteen studies. The reason for the drop in blood pressure is thought to be the efficacy of meditation in relaxing the large muscle groups surrounding the circulatory system. Meditation also relaxes the smaller muscles that control the blood vessels, which would effectively lower the pressure of the blood within them and compound the beneficial effect.

Many studies have consistently borne out these findings. In one study, patients using hypertensive drugs learned how to meditate using a mantra. Their average blood pressure dropped from 159/100 to 138/85 mmHg, much closer to the normal systolic pressure of 120–139 mmHg. In contrast, their counterparts with similar starting readings were told to relax on a couch for the same period of time. Their average blood pressure barely changed, from 163/99 mmHg to 162/97 mmHg.

Of course, meditation helps those who are not on drugs as well. In another study, half of the patients added 30 minutes of daily yogic breathing (*pranayama*) and muscle relaxation to their routines. The subjects who were not using hypertensive drugs reduced their blood pressure from an average of 134 mmHg to 107 mmHg. Those subjects who were using blood pressure medications had an average systolic BP drop from 120 mmHg to 110 mmHg—a noticeably lesser amount—even though they were taking medications.

As you might expect, meditation could be recommended to help prevent hypertension. And subjects with borderline hypertension in another study reported mean blood pressure reductions from 145/91 mmHg to 135/87 mmHg when they began meditating daily with a mantra. Most studies have also shown that blood pressure rates will revert to the higher readings if the regular practice of meditation is stopped.

Meditation and the Brain

As doctors have expanded their studies of the body and meditation's effects, a new science, called neurotheology, has emerged. Neurotheology is the study of how yoga, religion, and meditation affect the functioning of the brain. By studying yogis, Zen practitioners, Franciscan nuns, and serious practitioners of all faiths, scientists are learning which physical and chemical processes are affected by spiritual practices and meditation.

One recent study found evidence that daily meditation practice resulted in a thickening of the cerebral cortex, the area of the brain responsible for making decisions, focusing attention, and storing memory. Sara Lazar, a scientist at Massachusetts General Hospital, discovered recently that the brain's gray matter of twenty average men and women who meditated for 40 minutes per day was thicker than the gray matter of people who did not meditate. Her research also suggests that meditation slows the aging process of the brain.

Other interesting findings relate to the electrical waves that the human brain constantly emits. These waves can be measured in a laboratory, and different brain waves correlate to different psychophysical states of stress and/or relaxation. Alpha brain waves, among others, have long been known to reflect a relaxed, pleasurable state of mind and body. (The next time you sense you may be on the "same wavelength" as somebody else, you may be exactly right!)

In a study conducted in Japan in the 1960s, researchers studied the EEG readings of meditation masters and students. In meditation sessions, practitioners were observed progressing through four clearly delineated stages of brain-wave activity, with each stage reflecting reports of deepening relaxation. The stages were:

1. Characterized by the appearance of alpha waves

2. Characterized by an increase in amplitude of the alpha waves

3. Characterized by a decrease of alpha waves, leading to the appearance of rhythmical theta-wave trains (the final stage of relaxation).

In this study, the longer a person practiced meditation, the more pronounced the progression, intensity, and duration of the four stages.

According to Dr. David Wulff at Wheaton College in Massachusetts, the brain actually has a "spirituality circuit" that is activated by the practice of yoga and meditation. This circuit is related to areas in the prefrontal cortex—which deals with the quality of attention—and the middle and lower temporal lobe, which controls emotion, learning, and memory. Practicing meditation has been shown to reduce the amount of "noise" registered in the brain from both external stimuli and internal dialogue, and activate the areas of the brain that experience expansive emotional/psychological/spiritual states, such as joy, deep relaxation, and heightened awareness.

The science of neurotheology promises great advances in our understanding of higher human potentials, and it is in this area that much research is currently being done. All of this confirms the anecdotal evidence of meditators for hundreds of years, which holds that the regular practice of meditation has tremendous benefits for mental and physical health, and represents the cutting edge of both personal growth and human potential.

6

Meditations for Women

n the previous chapters we have discussed how to prepare your environment, body, and mind for the practice of meditation. We have examined many of the challenges women face and how meditation can help you meet those challenges. We have looked at scientific studies that explain how meditation benefits both body and mind. In the following pages, you will find some of the most powerful meditations taught by Yogi Bhajan. The meditations have been chosen to address a wide range of women's issues.

While all meditation practices can help you develop a relaxed and neutral mind and help you connect with your core identity, many meditation practices can target specific areas of your life. This is possible because of the endless combination of breath techniques, mudras, mantras, and visualizations.

Review the meditations in this section and choose a meditation that matches your present needs, interests, and level of experience. Practice this meditation at least three to five times, and then assess your experience. If you feel comfortable with the breath pattern, the mudra, and the mantra, and are beginning to notice positive effects from your practice, continue doing this meditation for forty days. The first benefits of meditation you will likely experience will be a noticeable feeling of relaxation and well-being after your meditation session. Although you may feel the benefits of meditation right away, it generally takes up to forty days to feel the more specific effects of each meditation and to notice its full impact.

 ## Meditation for Universal Wisdom

Gyan Mudra is called the mudra of wisdom. Meditating with your hands in *Gyan Mudra* while breathing deeply helps you experience universal wisdom and let go of confusion and doubt. Evaluate your mental state after three minutes of practice. You should find that you are more relaxed and focused. You can gradually build up this practice for longer periods.

Sit in a comfortable seated posture. Rest your hands on your knees, with your palms up or down. Curl your index fingers and capture the tips of their nails with the pad of the first joint of your thumbs—*Gyan Mudra*. The other three fingers of each hand are straight and close together. Hold your arms straight but not rigid, with no bend in the elbows. Your body is like a pyramid—balanced, symmetrical, and stable.

Inhale and exhale deeply through your nose. On your inhale feel as though you are pulling the breath down into your navel center.

Keep inhaling until your lungs have taken in all they can hold. Your chest will be expanded. When you exhale, empty the lungs completely. Keep track of the breath and feel it as it comes in and goes out. Make each inhalation and exhalation as long and full and complete as you can. As your breath slows down, the mind slows down also, and tends to put you to sleep. Stay alert and continue to make each breath full and deep. Consciously feel yourself taking in and absorbing universal wisdom with each inhalation, and getting rid of doubt and confusion with each exhalation. Continue for 3 minutes.

STAGES OF MEDITATION

 The stages of meditation are described as:

1. *Pratyahar*—In this stage you begin to bring your attention to the meditative process and synchronize your thoughts with your intention to remember your true identity during your meditation session.

2. *Dharana*—In this stage you develop the ability to hold your concentration on the meditation. Even as thoughts arise, you patiently and without strain continue to hold your mental focus.

3. *Dhyana*—In this stage you can enter into a deep meditative state. Your attention has fully and consistently shifted from the outer stimulations and distractions and begins to look steadily toward your true identity.

4. *Samadhi*—This is a profound state of existence. When you reach this stage, you have the constant experience of the fullness of your true identity and can live and act from that truth.

Meditation for Managing Stress

This is a basic technique in Kundalini Meditation. It is excellent to do before bed or when you want to distance yourself from the worries of the day. It can also reestablish emotional balance and calm after emotional shocks or after a period of intense stress. When practiced for 31 minutes, this technique can help you recover from past emotional trauma.

Sit in a meditative posture such as Easy Pose. Keep your spine relaxed and straight. Rest your left hand on your knee in *Gyan Mudra*. Close your eyes. Press the eyes up gently and focus at your Brow Point. Raise your right hand; palm is flat and faces to the left, in front of and to the right of your face. Block your right nostril with your thumb. Press just hard enough to close your nostril. Keep the rest of your fingers straight up (see photo, page 57). Inhale deeply through your left nostril. When your breath is full, release your thumb, bend your right hand into a U shape, and use the tip of your little fingertip to block your left nostril. Now, exhale smoothly, continuously, and completely through your right nostril. Then begin the cycle again with an inhalation through your left nostril. Continue with long deep regular breaths. Mentally chant the *Bij Mantra, Sat Naam,* in unison with your breath. Mentally chant *Sat* on your inhale and *Naam* on your exhale. Continue for 10–15 minutes. You can build up your practice of this meditation to 31 minutes. To end this meditation inhale, exhale completely and hold your breath out as you apply Root Lock, or *Mula Bandha* (see page 12). Inhale and relax completely.

Left Nostril Breathing for Relaxation, Receptivity, and a Peaceful Sleep

From a yogic perspective, the left nostril is associated with the moon and receptivity. When you breathe through the left nostril, you stimulate the part of your brain that is receptive. The result is a cooling and calming effect that helps you relax and rest. Practice left nostril breathing before bed for a restful sleep. Practice left nostril breathing if you are trying to call upon your receptive abilities to conceive a child.

Sit in a comfortable meditative posture with a straight spine. Relax your left hand in *Gyan Mudra* on your knee. Cover your right nostril with your right thumb and begin a slow and deep breath through your left nostril. Continue inhaling and exhaling through your left nostril. Continue breathing through your left nostril for 3–11 minutes. To end, inhale, suspend your breath briefly, and then relax.

Meditation into Being

This meditation uses the mantra I AM, I AM. The mantra I AM, I AM is common to many traditions. If you say to yourself, "I AM," the mind wants to know "I AM what?" Usually you follow I AM with words like happy, sad, good, bad, tall, short, and so on. When you replace these common responses with another I AM, your mind is directed to relate to infinity instead of the mundane identifications with emotions, the physical body, and desires. This meditation helps you build your true identity by reminding yourself that you are beyond any finite identification. This meditation can help young women begin to understand their true identity by lessening their attachment to their physical appearance and emotional fluctuations.

Sit in Easy Pose with the spine straight. Place your right hand in *Gyan Mudra* on your right knee. Hold your left hand facing your heart center about 6 inches from the chest. As you say I AM, bring your hand 4 inches in front of your chest (moving toward you). As you repeat I AM a second time, move your hand away from your body until it is 12 inches away from your chest. Take a short breath in as you return your hand to 6 inches from your chest. Continue this cycle for 3–11 minutes. You may gradually build up the time of this meditation to 31 minutes.

 Meditation for Total Relaxation

The following relaxation script was given by Yogi Bhajan to help you achieve deep physical and mental relaxation. Record the script in your own voice or read the words, meditate upon them, and then relax.

"Relax in total existence, relating under the total ordinance of your higher consciousness. Each cell of your body must relax. You are going to be a totally, extremely relaxed individual. Absolutely relax, relax with dignity, with perfect heart and consciousness and sweetness and beauty. Feel every cell of your body relaxing, deeper and deeper, steadier and steadier and steadier and steadier. Let everything go, let all the tension go. When you relax your body, God will prevail because of the *prana*—the energy of life—that gives you absolute health. O dear one, just relax, feel that the fingertips are falling away, the wrists are going away, everything is breaking. Shatter your body into all its cells, build it up, vibrate the aspects that are your basic elements of earth, water, fire, air, and ether or space."

Relax your earth element—your body—into the earth, relax all the blood and water in your body into the oceans, relax all the fiery element—your digestion, self will, and intensity into the fire of the sun, relax the air of your breath—and let it merge into the universal breath, relax the ether in you—your subtlety—and let it merge into the cosmos.

"Let your mind collaborate with you at this moment. Relax your body, your eyes, your eyebrows, your cheeks, your chin, your neck, your head, shoulders, rib cage, belly, and everything in it—waistline, thighs, shins, ankles, feet, toes, everything. Let the Divine flow through you. Allow yourself to receive It; every part of It is yours. It is your privilege, and you must have that privilege. Be extremely relaxed and use your mind to relax yourself. The ability to relax is the highest power of the self; therefore, please command yourself to relax. Become the master of the self, let this physical self obey your mental self and the *prana,* the soul, must prevail through you."

Meditation for Developing an Attitude of Gratitude

In this meditation, you simply sit and allow all the blessings of your life to fall into your cupped hands. Feel yourself merging with the light of those blessings. This meditation will help you awaken to and express your gratitude for the kindness and honest efforts of the people in your life.

Sit in Easy Pose with a straight spine. Bring your hands together approximately 6 inches from the front of your chest. Cup your

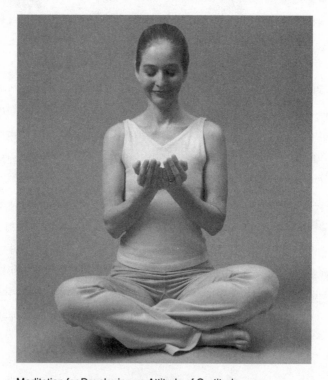

Meditation for Developing an Attitude of Gratitude

hands, with the edge of your right hand touching the edge of your left hand. Continue to hold the hand posture until you feel so relaxed that it seems even your eyelashes are relaxing.

 ## Meditation to Balance Behavior and Impulse

This meditation balances your behavior by balancing your energy flow. Life can be particularly stressful during the intense changes in hormone levels that accompany adolescence or menopause. This meditation can help you feel less emotional and out of control during these stressful transitions. It may take some time to build the discipline necessary to hold the posture, but the result is worth the effort!

Sit in Easy Pose with your spine straight. Place your hands, palms facing each other, at the level of your mouth. Keep your left wrist straight, and bend your right hand at the wrist. Your hands do not touch. The fingers of your right hand point down as the fingers of your left hand point up. Close your eyes and imagine you can see through your forehead. Sit in this posture for 3–11 minutes. After 3–11 minutes reverse your hands so the fingers of your right hand point up and the fingers of your left hand point down. Continue breathing normally in this posture for another 3–11 minutes, with 11 minutes per side being the ultimate goal.

KRIYA

A kriya is defined as a "complete action." These meditations are considered especially powerful and can be used daily or in times of special need.

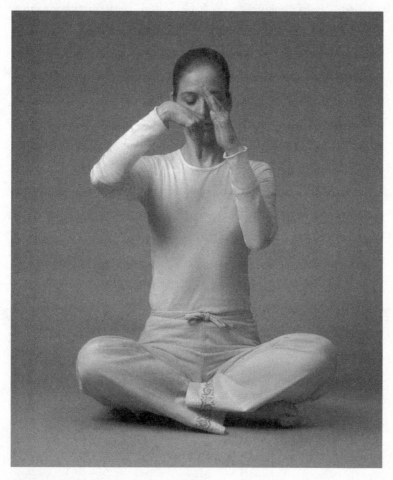

Meditation to Balance Behavior and Impulse

Sat Kriya for Total Elevation

If you only have a few minutes to practice Kundalini Yoga, do *Sat Kriya*. It is unmatched for increasing focus, concentration, and your core energy of awareness—the Kundalini. As you rhythmically pulse your navel area, you will strengthen your pelvic-floor muscles and stimulate your digestion. *Sat Kriya* synchronizes your mind, body, and soul, and creates new patterns of circulation throughout your entire system—both physically and energetically. *Sat Kriya* is effective in improving your mood and strengthening your individual projection, and it will help you to conquer chronic fears. And because this kriya awakens the energy of the first three chakras, you will have greater access to vitality, projection, and presence. Strengthening these qualities enables you to relax and stay centered.

Sit on your heels in Rock Pose. Clasp your hands together, keeping the index fingers extended. Stretch your arms straight up and over your head so that your elbows hug your ears. Cross your thumbs to hold your hands together and help you lock into the posture. Keep your elbows as straight as you can. Chant the mantra *Sat Naam* aloud with a powerful projection. As you chant *Sat,* pull your navel point in and up. You will feel your pelvic floor lift a bit. Do not flex your spine. As you chant *Naam,* release the navel point and relax your belly. Create a steady rhythm of about 8 *Sat Naam* repetitions per every 10 seconds. Concentrate on the mantra and the steady pulsing movement of your navel point area. Your breath will adjust itself. Continue for 3–11 minutes. To end the exercise, inhale deeply and hold the breath in without straining. Consciously apply the Root Lock, pulling in at the navel point and up on pelvic muscles, thus lifting the pelvic floor. Focus your eyes at your Brow Point. Hold for 5–10 seconds, and exhale. Repeat this sequence 2 more times, and then relax. After you complete *Sat Kriya,* it is best to relax for twice the amount of time that you practiced the exercise. This helps the energy stimulated by the exercise to become integrated into your body and mind.

Begin your practice for 1–3 minutes, and slowly build your time as your endurance and strength increase. One way to increase the time of *Sat Kriya* is to alternate 3 minutes of *Sat Kriya* with 3 minutes of rest. With common sense and a steady practice, you can gradually increase to 31 minutes.

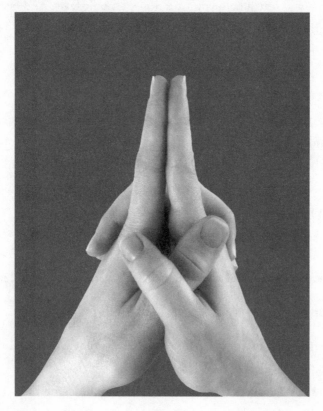

Mudra for *Sat Kriya*

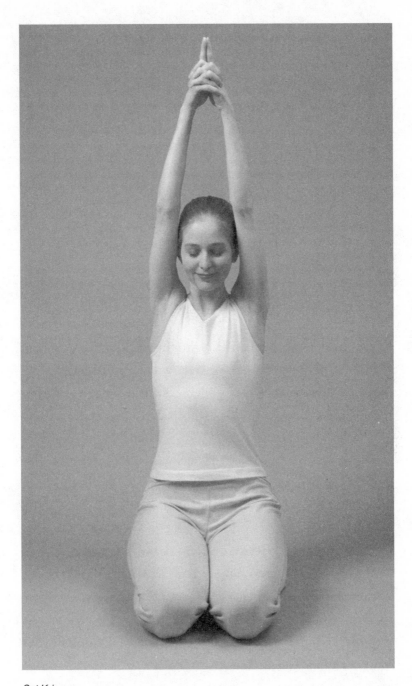

Sat Kriya

KUNDALINI ENERGY

 According to the philosophy of yoga, we all have an innate capacity for personal growth and self-realization. Kundalini energy can be described as an energy that lies dormant in all people. When it is awakened through meditation, yoga practice, or meaningful experiences in life, you feel empowered and have an experience of your core identity.

Kirtan Kriya for Mastering Your Moods

Kirtan Kriya is considered the highest meditation for a woman and should be a regular part of every woman's meditative practice. This meditation can help you break any habit and assist you in going through any transition or life change. *Kirtan Kriya* can also help in healing negative sexual memories and traumas. *Kirtan Kriya* can give a woman a brilliant internal radiance that illuminates her aura and presence. Physically, yogis believe *Kirtan Kriya* stimulates your pituitary and pineal glands to become active and balanced.

The mantra for both versions of *Kirtan Kriya, Saa Taa Naa Maa,* is called the *Panj Shabd,* which means the five sounds of life. These basic syllables are the primal sounds of the mantra *Sat Naam,* the seed mantra of Truth. The mantra *Saa Taa Naa Maa* reflects the wheel of life. Each sound creates a unique vibration in your body and mind. The meaning of this mantra is:

Saa—infinity, cosmos, beginning, and birth
Taa—life, existence
Naa—death, totality, and transition
Maa—rebirth, renewal

Version 1

Sit in Easy Pose or in a chair with your feet flat on the floor. Begin repeating the mantra *Saa Taa Naa Maa* aloud in a rhythmic way. Focus your eyes at your Brow Point. Imagine the sound current passing through your head in an L shape, entering through the crown (top) of your head and flowing out through the center of the forehead (Brow Point). As you chant *Saa,* press your index finger to the tip of your thumb; on *Taa,* press your middle finger to your thumb; on *Naa,* press your ring finger to your thumb; and on *Maa,* press your little finger to your thumb. Use enough pressure to really feel the connection. This helps keep you awake and in rhythm. Allow your breath to relax and regulate itself. Continue repeating the mantra aloud for 5 minutes. Then lower your voice to a whisper and continue repeating the mantra for 5 minutes. Next become silent and mentally repeat the mantra for 10 minutes. Keep using your fingers while you repeat the mantra silently. After 10 minutes of silent repetition, reverse the process, whispering for 5 minutes, and then repeat aloud for 5 minutes. Maintain the finger movements and mental imagery throughout. To end the meditation, inhale and exhale deeply as you stretch your arms up as far as possible, spreading your fingers wide, for 1 minute. Then relax.

Beginners may want to shorten the time to 2 to 3 minutes for each cycle of chanting (aloud-whisper-silent), then build gradually to the full 31 minutes. With patience, dedication, and common sense, you can build this meditation to 2½ hours.

The finger movements balance your brain and the different qualities of your personality. Each time you touch your finger to your thumb, for instance, you balance and integrate the qualities of infinity, beginning, and birth into your whole being.

When you chant aloud, you relate to the realm of the earth and to humanity. When you whisper, you relate to the realm of lovers, longing to belong and relate. When you chant silently, you relate to the realm of the Divine and of Infinity, beyond time and space. By chanting in all three voices, you can achieve a harmonious balance in body, mind, and soul.

Version 2

Lie on your stomach and place your chin on the floor. Keep your head straight, without looking left or right. Place your arms alongside your body, with the palms of the hands facing upward.

Begin to mentally chant the *Panj Shabd, Saa Taa Naa Maa.* Focus your eyes at your Brow Point. Use the same L-shaped energy circuit and the same finger motions with the silently chanted mantra as in Version 1.

Continue in this manner for 3 to 31 minutes. This posture places the head and neck in an uncommon position, so start slowly and rest your head to one side if your neck becomes stiff.

Kirtan Kriya chanted in the belly position with your chin on the floor balances your Moon Centers, particular centers of energetic focus in women. For an in-depth discussion of Moon Centers, see my previous book, coauthored with Dr. Machelle Seibel, *A Woman's Book of Yoga.*

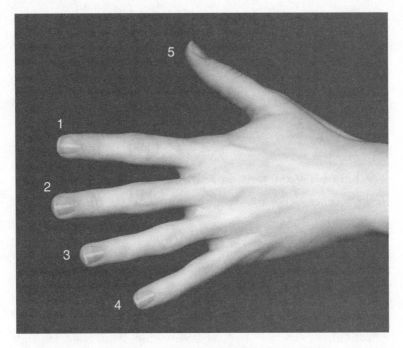

The Power of Mudra—The Qualities Associated with Each Finger

1. Index Finger—Jupiter finger: knowledge and expansion

2. Middle Finger—Saturn finger: patience, transforming emotions to devotion, responsibility

3. Ring Finger—Sun finger: physical vitality, health, beauty

4. Little Finger—Mercury finger: communication, functioning in the world

5. Thumb: positive ego

Karani Kriya for Stablizing Your Core Identity

The practice of this *kriya* can help you break the habit of looking outside yourself for approval, thus enabling you to stabilize your core identity. This *kriya* can also help you maintain your core identity amid the many roles you play throughout your life (mother, wife, businessperson). This meditation empowers the energy center located at your throat that gives you the power of disciplined speech and wise communication.

Sit in Easy Pose with your spine straight. Extend your arms straight out to the sides of your body, parallel to the ground, with your elbows bent. Draw your hands in toward your chest until they meet in front of your chest at the level of your chin. Bend your ring and little fingers under your hands and hold them in place with your thumbs. Point the extended fingers at each other with the fingertips touching. Be sure to keep your arms parallel to the ground. Your eyes are slightly (one-tenth) open. Begin the following breath pattern:

Deeply inhale for 2–3 seconds. Suspend your breath for 5 seconds. Exhale slowly for 10–15 seconds, making sure you completely exhale.

Continue this breath rhythm for 11 minutes. To end, inhale deeply, exhale, and relax.

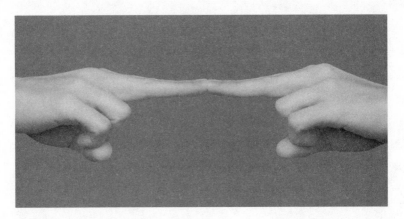

Mudra for *Karani Kriya*

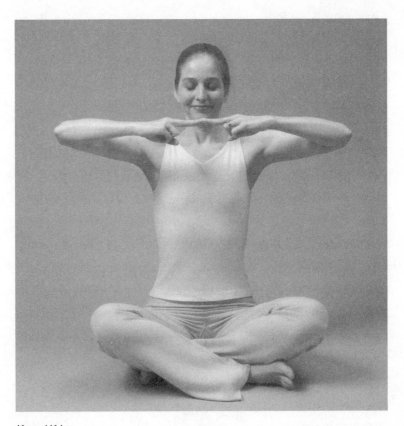

Karani Kriya

Rejuvenation Meditation

This meditation can be considered a medical meditation. While it does not replace allopathic forms of medicine, its effects can be considered strong enough to help your system fight disease. This meditation can positively affect your glandular system, stimulating your natural capacity to heal. It is best to do before going to bed. With practice you can feel the profound effects breath control has on your mind and body.

Sit in Easy Pose. Relax your arms down along your sides. Bring your hands up in front of your chest with your palms toward your torso. Keep your elbows snug against the side of your ribs. Join your hands along the sides of your palms and your little fingers. Spread your fingers and thumbs apart and bend your wrists so your palms face up toward the sky, making a bowl shape.

Focus your eyes past the tip of your nose toward the distant ground and beyond into the depths of the earth.

Begin the following breath pattern; it should be done precisely. Inhale deeply and slowly through semi-puckered lips. Hold the breath in for 4 seconds (the length of one mental repetition of *Saa Taa Naa Maa.* Then exhale, powerfully in 4 equal strokes through the nose. As you exhale, mentally recite the mantra *Saa Taa Naa Maa.* Then hold the breath out for 2 seconds (or the length of one mental repetition of *Wha-hay Guroo*). Continue this meditation for 11 minutes. With practice you can extend it to 31 minutes. Start slowly with this breathing pattern, as it can make you feel spacey and dreamy. Begin your practice with 3 minutes if it is appropriate for you.

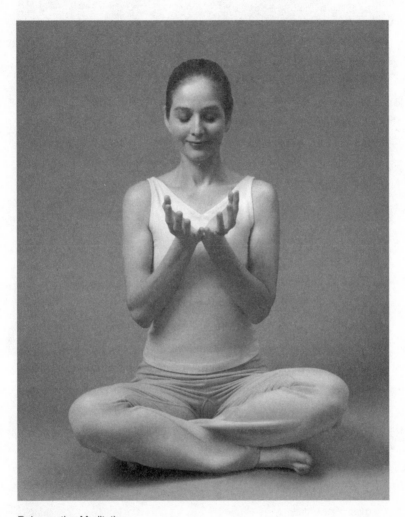

Rejuvenation Meditation

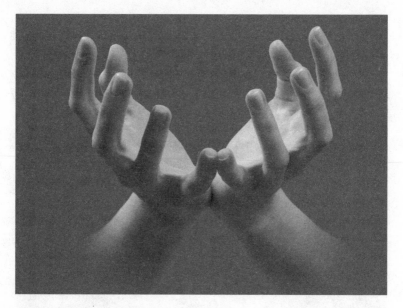

Mudra for Rejuvenation Meditation

A MANTRA FOR ECSTASY
AND REMEMBRANCE

Wha-hay Guroo is a powerful mantra that is commonly used in Kundalini Meditation as taught by Yogi Bhajan. It is considered the mantra of ecstasy and of dwelling in your infinite identity. The repetition of this mantra is said to remind your soul of its true nature.

A Movement Meditation to Release Physical and Mental Stress

Some meditations include movement. Rhythmic, unforced, graceful, and free movements can help release tension stored in the body. Emotional traumas can leave their signatures of tension in your body. If these areas of the body are not relaxed, chronic stress can take hold and lead to both physical and mental imbalances. Feeling your entire body confirms the reality of your newly relaxed state and calms your aura. The next exercises strengthen your heart and circulatory system. This simple series is for total relaxation of body and mind. The time of the first exercise can be extended as long as you enjoy it. In a normal session, 3–5 minutes is enough.

Part 1

Stand straight with your arms completely relaxed. Close your eyes. Feel any tension in each part of your body and consciously let it go. Next, begin to sway and move every part of your body. Dance gracefully. Feel the easy movement of each body area. If there is gentle rhythmic music of a high vibration available, it may be used as a background. Continue for 3–11 minutes.

Part 2

Immediately stand straight with your eyes still closed. With your hands, begin to lightly feel each part and area of your body without reservation. Every square inch must be touched. Feel sensitively with the palms. Continue for 3–5 minutes.

Part 3

Standing Forward Bend (*Uttanasana*). Lean forward with your arms hanging completely relaxed. All the muscles of your body should relax. Let the breath be normal. Continue for 3–11 minutes.

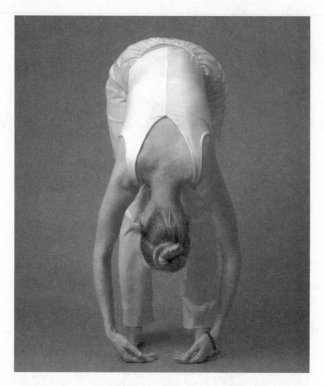

Standing Forward Bend (*Uttanasana*)

Part 4

Standing Backward Bend (*Utthitardha-Chakrasana*). Inhale and exhale deeply several times. Next, slowly lean back with your arms hanging loosely down. Breathing is relaxed. Hold for 1 minute. Completely relax.

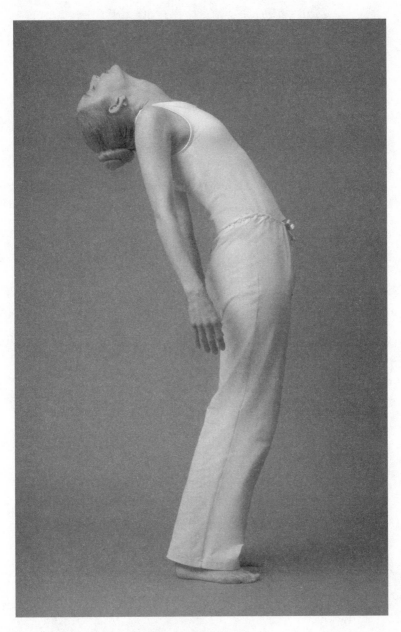

Standing Backward Bend (*Utthitardha-Chakrasana*)

Antar Naad Mantra Kriya Meditation— Celestial Communication

The practice of this mantra can help your creativity flow and spark your imagination. This mantra helps stimulate total balance through energizing the chakras—the energy centers from the base of your spine to the crown of your head. This meditation is a good place to start if you want to understand the deeper effects of chanting and sound. This meditation has two versions. Both versions use the *Antar Naad Mantra:*

Saa Ray Saa Saa Saa Ray Saa Saa Saa Ray Saa Saa Saa Rung
Har (a) Ray, Har (a) Har (a), Har (a) Ray, Har (a) Har (a),
Har (a) Ray, Har (a) Har (a), Har (a) Rung

This mantra encompasses the creativity of the Kundalini—the transforming energy of life. *Saa* means the infinite, representing the subtle element and quality of ether. Chanting *Saa* stimulates your subtlety and grace. *Har* is the creativity of the earth. It is the power of manifestation, the tangible and the personal. By chanting *Saa* and *Har* in a rhythm, you can achieve a balance between your subtlety and your earthiness. The sounds of *Har* and *Saa* are woven together with the sound of *Ung* which refers to complete totality, like the mantra *Ong* or *Aum.*

Version 1: Experiencing the Essence of Sound and Mantra

Sit in Easy Pose. Keep the spine straight. Let the arms extend straight and rest over the knees. Make *Buddhi Mudra* with both hands: Touch your thumb tips to the tips of your little fingers. Your other fingers are straight but relaxed. Become completely still, physically and mentally, like a calm ocean. Listen to, or mentally chant, the mantra for 1 minute. Feel its rhythm in every cell. Then begin to chant it aloud. Continue for 11–31 minutes.

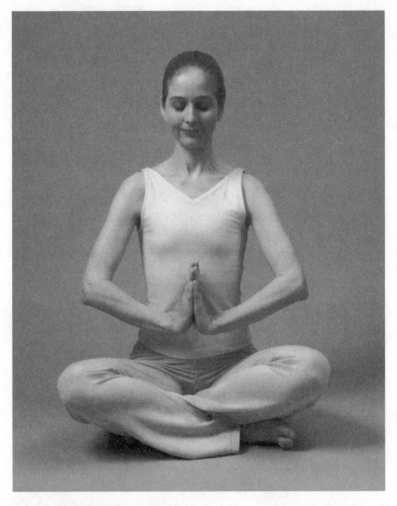

Celestial Communication, starting position

Version 2: Balance and Creativity

The particular moving mudra in this meditation is a key to opening the flow of Kundalini—a state of increased awareness. This new awareness gives you a direct experience of your true self.

CELESTIAL COMMUNICATION

Celestial Communication is an easy and effective meditation technique. You can listen to any beautiful and inspiring mantra music and, while sitting in a meditative posture, allow your upper body to dance. Move your arms, hands, fingers, and torso to the music. You can create your own movements that repeat with the mantra, and be as creative as you like. Try to allow your body to respond to the mantra and the music, instead of trying to intellectually create a dance. This form of meditation is appropriate for all ages; children and young women especially love it.

The initial movement in this celestial communication involves a slow transition between Prayer Pose, or *Atmanjali Mudra* (palms flat together) and Open Lotus. Open Lotus is formed by touching the base of your palms together while also connecting the tips of your little fingers together and the tips of your thumbs together. The rest of your fingers are spread open.

Put your hands in a Prayer Pose (*Atmanjali Mudra*) at the level of your navel point. As the mantra starts with *Saa Ray Saa Saa,* begin to raise your hands up the centerline of your torso, about

4–6 inches out in front of your body. As your hands pass your heart center, begin to open them, like a blooming flower, into Open Lotus. Time your motion so that your hands are in full Open Lotus at the level of your brow point on the sound *Saa Rung*.

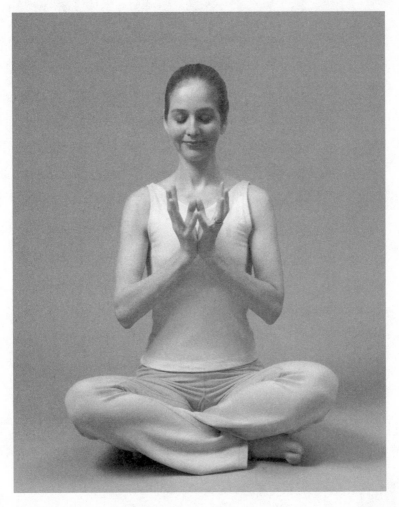

Celestial Communication, as your arms move upward

As the mantra begins *Har Ray Har Har,* turn the fingers to point down, with the back of the hands touching—this is Reverse Prayer Pose. Slowly bring this mudra back down the centerline of your body until your fingertips reach your navel point on the sounds *Ha Rung.* Then turn them around and begin again.

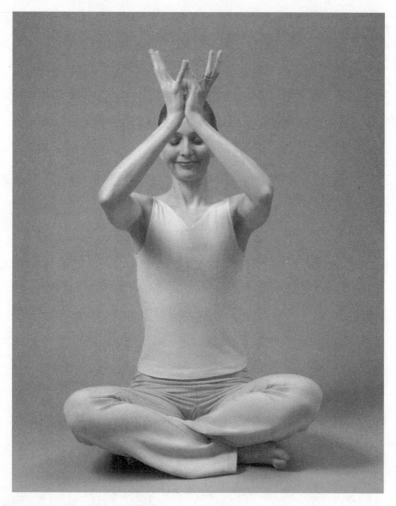

Celestial Communication, as your hands reach your brow point

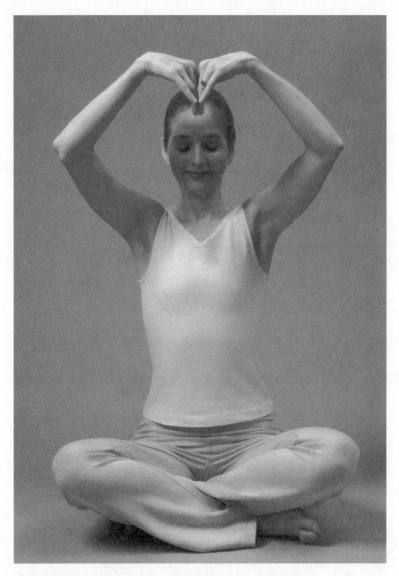

Celestial Communication, as your hands begin to move downward

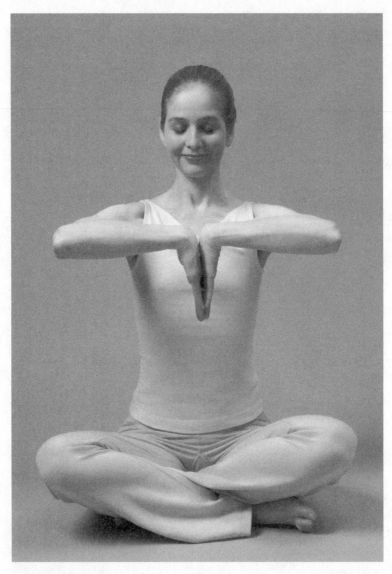

Celestial Communication, as your arms move downward in front
of the heart center

Divine Shield Meditation— Building Strength and Security

It can be difficult to live in your true identity if you feel fearful and unprotected. One way to feel more secure is to strengthen your aura by using an inner seed sound that activates the power of the heart center. When you expand your heart energy in this way, your aura becomes stronger. It provides a divine shield to accompany you through your life experiences.

THE AURA

The aura can be described as your energetic projection and your energetic protection, and includes the space around your body in all directions. If your aura is healthy, it can extend to as much as nine feet from your body! A healthy aura helps you filter out and cut through negativity, and helps you hold your identity in the midst of surrounding confusion or the negativity of others. One of the best things a woman can do is to develop her aura. Certain meditations, yoga exercises, and breathing techniques are specifically designed to help build a woman's aura.

This meditation uses the mantra *Ma*. The sound of *Ma* is a sound of the heart. This sound calls on compassion and protection. It is the same sound that a baby uses to call on the mother. In this case, your soul is the child and the universe becomes the mother. If you call, the universe will come to your aid and comfort.

Sit in Easy Pose. Raise your right knee up so your right foot is flat on the ground with the toes pointing straight ahead. Place the sole of your left foot against the arch and ankle of your right foot. The ball of your left foot rests just in front of the anklebone of your right foot.

Make your left hand into a fist and place it on the ground beside your left hip. Use it to balance your posture. Place your right elbow on the top of your right knee and bring your right hand back along the side of your head. With the palm facing the ear, bring the right hand back along the side of the head. Form a shallow cup of the right palm. Then bring it against the skull so that it makes contact below the ear, but stays open above the ear. It is as if you cupped your hand to amplify a faint sound that you want to hear.

Close your eyes and focus them at your Brow Point. Inhale deeply and chant the sound *Maaaaaaaaa*. Chant it at a comfortable high pitch with a long, full smooth sound. Project the sound as if someone were listening to you. As you chant, listen to the sound and let it vibrate through your whole body. If you chant in a group, hear the overtones that develop and let those tones vibrate all around you and in every cell of your body. When you have exhaled completely, take another deep breath and continue. Hold your concentration on the sound current. In a group you may all inhale at different times, and the resulting sound will seem continuous. Continue for 11–31 minutes. Then switch sides and continue for an equal amount of time. When first practicing this meditation, start slowly, meditating for 3 minutes on each side.

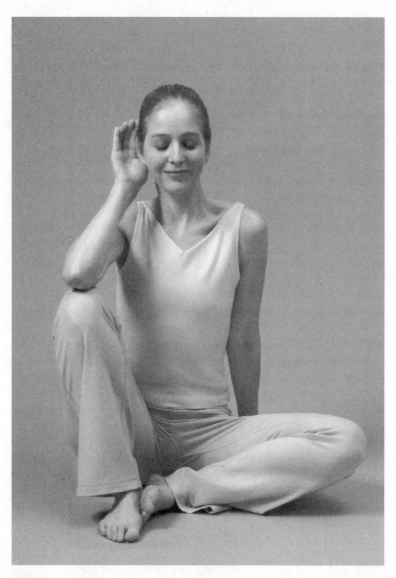

Divine Shield Meditation

Meditation to Make You Feel Cozy and Contented

The practice of this meditation can make you feel cozy and contented, and at the same time strengthen your nervous system if you are facing hard times ahead.

Sit in Easy Pose. Connect the tips of your thumb and middle finger of your right hand, and the tips of your thumb and little finger of your left hand (males would reverse this posture). The fingernails in this mudra do not touch. Position your hands a little in front of your chest at the height of your nipples. Hold your hands 7–8 inches apart from each other, with your palms facing upward and elbows out to the sides. Allow your shoulders to relax. Keep your eyes slightly (one-tenth) open. Allow your breath to be relaxed and natural. Continue for 3–11 minutes. To end, inhale and make tight fists with both of your hands for a few seconds, and then relax.

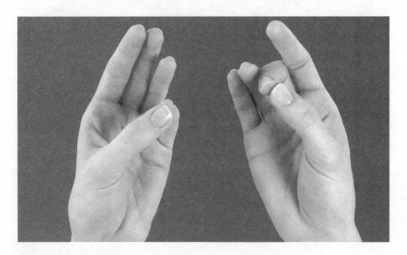

Mudra for Meditation to Make You Feel Cozy and Contented

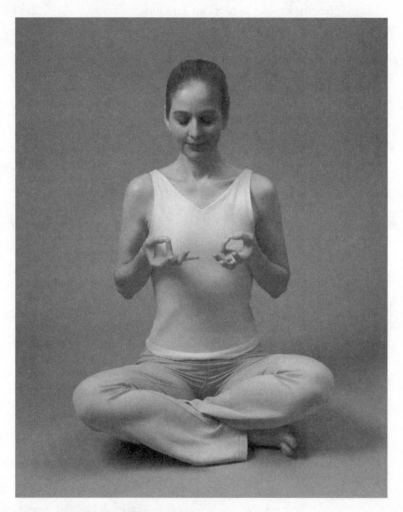

Meditation to Make You Feel Cozy and Contented

Meditation to Deal with Frustration

This meditation has three parts and includes some yoga postures. Practice this meditation when you are experiencing feelings of frustration. This meditation is effective because of the combination and sequence of these postures. First, meditating in the posture with your spine stretched, as in the first part of this meditation (Part 1), creates a natural balance to the glandular system—particularly your thyroid and parathyroid. As you hold the posture, a certain area of the brain will open. This section of the brain supports your efforts to let go of your frustration. Next, Baby Pose, or *Mudhasana,* promotes deep relaxation and security (Part 2). When you practice it you stimulate the flow of *prana*—life-giving energy—to the areas of the brain that opened during the previous part of the meditation. And, finally, when you laugh at the end of the meditation, you empower your intention to let go and lighten up (Part 3). Laughter stimulates the energy of the navel point.

Part 1:

Come onto the floor on your hands and knees. Place your hands directly below your shoulders and your knees directly below your hips. Arch your spine downward, letting your belly drop toward the floor, and allow your head to rise up so that your eyes are looking at the sky. Keep your head in alignment with your spine so your spine is in a graceful upward curve. Hold your head as high as you can comfortably and fix your eyes on one point on the sky above you. Hold this posture and begin Long Deep Breathing.

For 1 minute simply follow the flow of your breath. Then

begin the following mental exercise: Think of something that is bothering you or bring up any thought that you would like to release. Start mentally wrestling with the issue. This is called churning of the mental self. Remain steady in the posture, keeping your head back, and continue wrestling with the issue for 7 minutes.

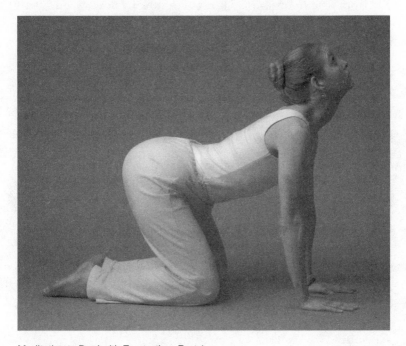

Meditation to Deal with Frustration, Part 1

Part 2:

Now sit back on your heels in Rock Pose and touch your forehead to the ground. This posture is Baby Pose, or *Mudhasana*. Allow your hands to rest by your sides, with palms facing up. You can place a pillow under your head if it does not rest comfortably on the floor. Relax in this posture. Let all tension drain from you. Allow infinite love to continually flow to you as you relax. Continue for 4–5 minutes.

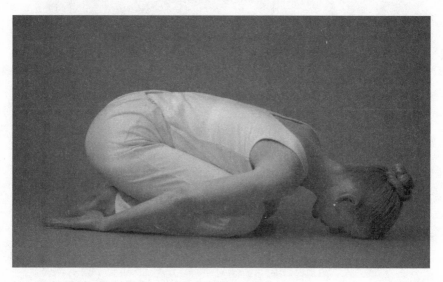

Meditation to Deal with Frustration, Part 2

Part 3:

Finally, rise up slowly so you are sitting on your heels and begin to laugh! Look at the sky and laugh.

Note: Baby Pose is an inverted posture. If you have high or low blood pressure or if you feel undue pressure on your head, use a pillow under it for support.

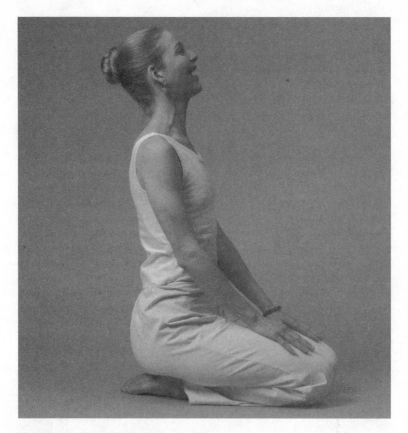

Meditation to Deal with Frustration, Part 3

 ## Meditation to Get Rid of Unwanted Sexual Desire

Sexual energy is a powerful force that is natural to a woman's life. Sexual energy can be transformed into creative energy that can supply fuel for all kinds of creative endeavors. However, sexual energy can also be so strong that it can distract a woman from her inner values and stability. This meditation can help you relax and focus when your sexual energy is distracting you.

Sit in Easy Pose or any comfortable cross-legged posture. Raise your arms to a 60-degree angle and tilt your head back. Open your mouth and flare your nostrils. Open yourself to the universe. Make the sound of *ahhhhhhhhhhhhhhh* 3 or 4 times. Then inhale, exhale, and relax. This meditation takes just a few minutes.

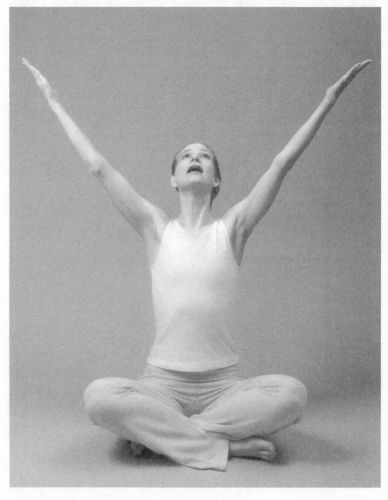

Meditation to Get Rid of Unwanted Sexual Desire

Meditation to Conquer Inner Anger and Burn It Out

This meditation can help you release even the most deeply seated anger. Unresolved anger can be the source of destructive thought patterns and fears that can negatively affect your physical health and your mental well-being. Choosing to practice this meditation is one way to make the commitment to let go of anger. Your index finger—Jupiter Finger—represents the quality of wisdom and expansion. Holding this finger straight and stiff can bring you extra support for living from wisdom and truth, thus facilitating the release of your anger. In this meditation you roll your tongue; rolling the sides of your tongue toward each other and creating a channel through which you inhale. You exhale through your nose. This is a breathing technique called *Sitali Pranayam,* which helps to cool the heat of anger. Rolling the tongue in this manner can be difficult for some women. If you cannot roll the tongue, simply pucker your lips and stick your tongue out about an inch outside of your mouth. Inhale the cool breath through your puckered lips and over the tongue.

Sit in Easy Pose. Extend both of your arms out straight to the sides and parallel to the ground, with no bend in your elbows. Point your index finger upward, pointing to the sky, while your thumb holds down your other fingers into a light fist. Keep the index fingers straight and stiff. Close your eyes and concentrate on your spine. Inhale deeply through your rolled tongue and exhale through the nose. Continue for up to 11 minutes.

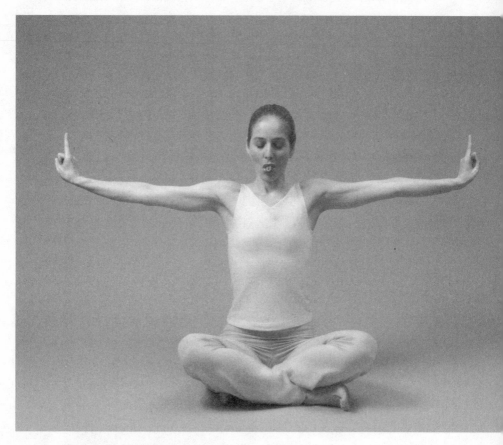

Meditation to Conquer Inner Anger and Burn It Out

Simple Meditation to Overcome Feeling Crazy

Do this meditation anytime you are feeling crazy or out of control. The fine motor control movements will help you feel more balanced and relaxed.

Sit in Easy Pose. Your upper arms are parallel to the ground with your forearms and fingers pointing toward the sky. Spread your fingers and rotate your hands back and forth, pivoting at the wrist. Continue this motion for 5 minutes.

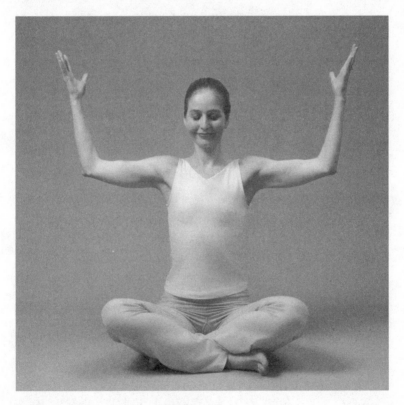

Simple Meditation to Overcome Feeling Crazy

Meditation for Love Without Attachment, for Kindness, Forgiveness, Sweetness, and Knowing That God Is Within You

This meditation uses the power of visualization to help you feel light and happy, and to create a sense of inner strength. With a strong inner light, you can communicate from your heart and bring honesty to your relationships. You may find it difficult to do this when you are feeling negative, but if you persevere and simply repeat the words aloud, or read them, you can change your mental state. If you repeat these words often enough, they become part of your reality.

Before you do this meditation, you may want to record the verbal part of the meditation, or have a friend read it to you. If you read it often, you may memorize it!

Sit in Easy Pose. Place your left hand in *Gyan Mudra* and rest it on your left knee with your arm straight. Use your right thumb to cover your right nostril and begin to breathe deeply through your left nostril. Concentrate at the top of your head. Take a vow for yourself:

After this day, if I have had any negativity toward any soul, consciously or unconsciously, I now forgive and I am kind to the whole universe. I am I am and I am a kind being. I am I am I am a beautiful being, a great being, a truthful being. Kindness and love. I am filled with it. That is what I am. All love, all kindness, all love, all sweetness, all sweetness, all smiles. I am I am. I came to go, I go to come. I am a free being. I don't want any attachments. Attachments will make me heavy. I want to be light. I am I am I am very light, light,

light, lighter than a feather, lighter than a rose petal, lighter than anything in this room, lightest of the light, lighter than light, completely light. I am a living truth. I am a living reality. God is within me. Let me go within and see God. God is in me and let me go within and see God. God the Creator, the Creator of the universe. That is what I am. I am pure, pure, pure manifestation of God.

Now inhale, exhale, and relax. The time of this meditation is simply however long it takes to speak it.

 ## *Pikhna Bhaki:* Meditation to See the Divine in Your Partner or Others

This can be an enjoyable devotional meditation. Any time you want to let go of grudges or blame, inspire yourself with the wisdom of others, or simply feel your natural compassion and love, practice this beautiful meditation.

Sit in Easy Pose. Close your eyes and focus them toward the tip of your nose. Imagine the back of your closed eyes is a movie screen and project a picture of anyone you know well—husband, holy person, deity, friend, teacher. Relax and meditate on the figure you've created in your mind. Continue as long as is comfortable—the time for this meditation is open.

Meditation to Awaken Compassion

When you feel tired or stressed and you feel there is no compassion left in your heart, this meditation can provide a healing spark to help ignite your inner light. Pregnancy and raising a family, building a career, or caring for parents or loved ones can be exhausting. This meditation can help you to replenish your energy so you can bring renewed compassion into your relationships. However, practicing this meditation can be compared to drinking sweet nectar. Overdrinking nectar can sometimes upset your stomach! So just do it 3 to 7 minutes in absolute calmness.

The mantra for this meditation is called the *Chotay Pad Mantra:*

Sat Naarayan Wha-hay Guroo
Haree Naarayan Sat Naam

Naarayan is the aspect of infinity that relates to the element of water, and *Haree Naarayan* is the Creative Sustainer. This mantra is related closely with the heart center and can cleanse the mind of all negativity. A person with chronic low self-esteem can become majestic by chanting this mantra. This meditation can provide a feeling of release and deep healing that can lead to the experience of clear and intuitive states of mind. To do this meditation, simply read the mantra, or chant in the melody provided.

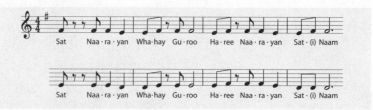

Musical Notation for *Chotay Pad Mantra*

Sit in Easy Pose with a straight spine. Hold your right hand in *Gyan Mudra* with the index finger curled under the thumb and the other fingers straight and joined together. Rest this hand on your right knee. With your left elbow bent and relaxed near your body, place your left hand about 6 inches in front of your heart center with your palm facing your body. The fingers and thumb are together and joined. To be effective, the fingers and the fingertips have to be held straight and totally tense. Concentrate on the hand as a shield to the heart. Inhale deeply and then exhale deeply. Repeat twice more, then inhale and begin chanting the mantra.

Continue to chant for 3–7 minutes. As you concentrate on the shield of the hand, you may feel the heat of powerful energy going through the hand to the heart center.

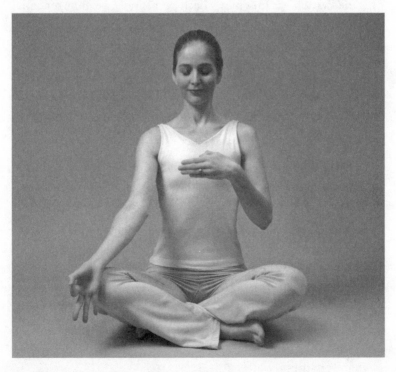

Meditation to Awaken Compassion

Kundalini Bhakti Mantra: Meditation on the Divine Mother, *Adi Shakti*

This meditation gives the power of concentration. It tunes you in to the primal, protective, and generating energy in the cosmos. This meditation can eliminate fear and can fulfill the longings of your heart. It gives you the power to act by removing the insecurities that block action. Practicing this meditation can also help heal feelings of loss and abandonment regarding our biological mothers, and help women connect with the universal and archetypal Mother.

This meditation has four parts. Each part should be done for equal lengths of time. They can be practiced for 11, 31, or 62 minutes.

Part 1:

Sit in Easy Pose with your hands in *Gyan Mudra,* resting on your knees. Imagine a spiral. This will represent the primal womb. Close your eyes and place this image in your mind's eye. Meditate on the infinite energy coming from the primal womb, an unending spiral, without beginning or end, going to infinity.

Part 2:

With your eyes still closed, put your hands 4 to 6 inches in front of your face with your palms facing each other. Cup your hands a little bit to make a circle of them, but leave them apart. Begin to mentally beam the spiral energy out through your hands to infinity.

Part 3:

Go deeper into meditation. Keep your hands fixed in place. Let your breath become long, deep, and slow. Begin to chant *Saa Taa Naa Maa* slowly as you exhale. Put your mind into the infinite light.

Part 4:

Continue to hold the posture and mental imagery and begin to chant the *Kundalini Bhakti Mantra*, pronounced as follows:

Aadee Shaktee, Aadee Shaktee, Aadee Shaktee, Namo Namo
Sarab Shaktee, Sarab Shaktee, Sarab Shaktee, Namo Namo
Prithum Bagvatee, Prithum Bagvatee,
Prithum Bagvatee, Namo Namo
Kundalini Maat Shaktee, Maat Shaktee, Namo Namo

Aadee Shaktee—the primal power

Sarab Shaktee—all power

Prithum Bagvatee—which creates through Infinite Love and Divine Light

Kundalini Maat Shaktee—*Kundalini,* the Mother Power

Namo—I bow down to, recognize

When a woman chants the mantra the Universal Energy will serve her. Break the barrier of intellect—let your heart open up to infinity. Nothing can come between *atma* (Soul) and *paramatma* (Universal Soul) when there is love.

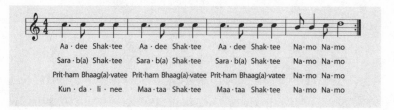

Musical Notation for *Kundalini Bhakti Mantra*

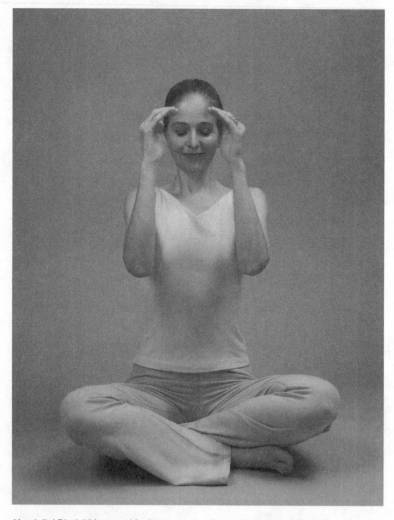

Kundalini Bhakti Mantra—Meditation on the Divine Mother, *Adi Shakti*

Meditation for Projection and Protection

This meditation is a celestial communication that builds your aura, arc line, and projection, giving you strength and self-confidence. With self-confidence comes the ability to communicate honestly and from the heart. This meditation uses a mantra called the *Mangala Charn Mantra*. It is a vibration that reaches deep into the archives of ancient wisdom. Here is the basic meaning of the words:

Aad Guray Nameh	*I bow to Primal Wisdom*
Jugaad Guray Nameh	*I bow to the Wisdom through the Ages*
Sat Guray Nameh	*I bow to the True Wisdom*
Siree Guroo Dayv-ay Nameh	*I bow to the great, unseen Wisdom*

The concept of bowing is common in many yoga traditions. When you encounter the word *bow* or the posture in yoga, think about the physical movement of bowing. When you bow, your heart is higher than your head. When you bow to wisdom, you are affirming that the wisdom of the heart will lead you, not your random thoughts.

Sit in Easy Pose. Place your palms together at your heart center in Prayer Pose, or *Atmanjali Mudra*. Your thumbs are crossed, left thumb over right (reverse for men). Chant the mantra and move your arms as indicated:

Aad Guray Nameh
Extend your arms in front of you and up
toward the sky at a 60-degree angle.

Jugaad Guray Nameh
Return your arms to Prayer Pose at your heart center.

Sat Guray Nameh
Extend your arms up and out again.

Siree Guroo Dayv-ay Nameh
Return your arms to your heart center again.

Chanting and movements occur together. As you chant, project
your mind and fully stretch your arms. Continue the meditation
for 11 minutes. As you perfect the meditation, extend the time in
5-minute intervals up to a maximum practice of 31 minutes.

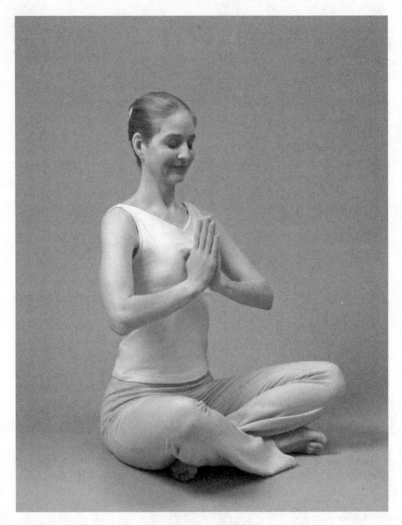

Meditation for Projection and Protection from the Heart, step one

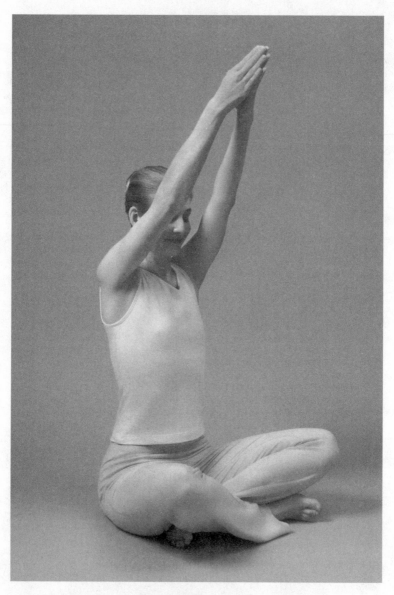

Meditation for Projection and Protection from the Heart, step two

Meditation for the Blossoming of Your True Self

This simple meditation is extremely relaxing. When you feel worried or stressed, take a moment to call on your inner resources using this meditation, and feel exalted.

Sit in a comfortable meditative posture with a straight spine. Bring your hands in front of your throat center. Place the base of your palms together and form your hands into the shape of a flower in full bloom. Your fingers will open and spread apart and your hands will be cupped. Now, keeping the base of your palms touching, gently allow your fingertips and thumb tips to touch, as if closing the flower, and then open again as if the flower is once again blooming. Continue opening and closing the flower. Close your eyes and feel "I am infinity. I am the rose." Feel as if you are blossoming, opening up.

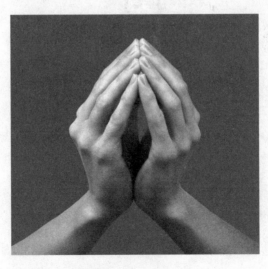

Lotus *Mudra* for the Blossoming of Your
True Self—Closed Lotus

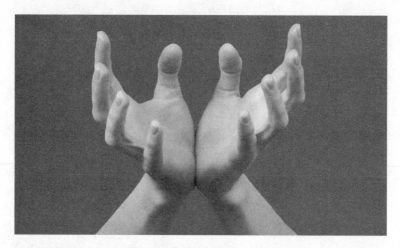

Lotus *Mudra* for the Blossoming of Your True Self—Open Lotus

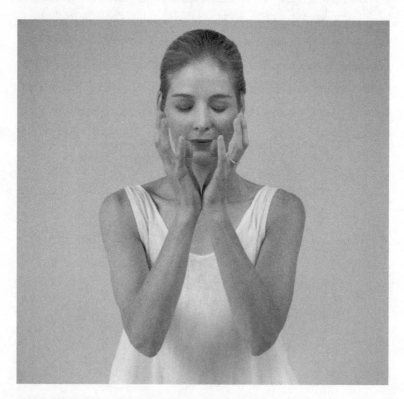

Meditation for the Blossoming of Your True Self

Meditation to Develop the Power of Your Word

Here are the comments Yogi Bhajan made regarding this meditation:

> The moment you start calming yourself, many negative thoughts may begin to surface. Some thoughts can be surprising or disturbing at times. Keep repeating the mantra. Cut through the negative thoughts with the mantra. Within 11 or 22 or 31 minutes your intellect will give up. The negative thoughts will cease to distract you. You can then enjoy the mantra and the state of mental relaxation that comes from conquering your own mind. This meditation can bring you an awareness of how important your words are, how they affect your mind, how they affect others, and how they create your world.

Sit comfortably with a straight spine. Relax your hands on your knees in *Gyan Mudra*. No eye focus is given, so allow your eyes to be comfortable—closed is a good choice. You may choose any mantra listed here or another mantra that speaks to you. Allow your breath to relax. Focus your mind on the mantra you choose and simply mentally repeat the mantra. Allow any negative thoughts to be diffused by the repetition of the mantra. Continue for as long as you like, until you start to enter a state of mental relaxation. Suggested times are 11, 22, or 31 minutes.

Some mantras to choose from:

Sat Naam—True Name—True Identity

Wha-hay Guroo—Mantra of ecstasy

Har Haray Haree Wha-hay Guroo—Har is like the seed, *Haray* is like the stem of the plant, and *Haree* is like the fragrance and color of the plant. If you balance these aspects of yourself, you can experience the ecstasy of that balance.

*Saa Taa Naa Maa—*The mantra of the cycle of life, birth, death, or transition, rebirth, and renewal. This mantra can help you through the transitions of life.

"Healthy am I, Happy am I, Holy am I"—an uplifting mantra in English!

 ## Meditation for Creating Caliber— Living Life with Full Expression, Accomplishment, and Success

This meditation will help you maintain your core identity under stress. It stimulates your inner resources, giving you a sense of expansiveness and the confidence to live from your destiny and inner truth instead of your fear. Meditating with your eyes open may be a new experience for you. The yogis link the eye postures in yoga to the optic nerve and then, ultimately, to the activity of the brain. When you meditate with your eyes open, you may feel your vision getting cloudy, or expanded, as if your peripheral vision is increasing. This is a common experience. If you find this uncomfortable, just close your eyes for a moment, relax your eyes, and open them when you feel ready to focus again.

Sit in Easy Pose with a straight spine. With both of your elbows relaxed by the sides of your body, raise your right hand up to the level of your face. Hold your fingers straight together and pointed straight up with your thumb relaxed, and your palm facing to the left. Bring your left hand up with your palm facing your body and your fingers pointed to the right. Hold your fingers together with the thumb pointing up. The tip of the middle finger of your left hand touches your right palm. Hold this mudra so that you first look right over the index finger, then slowly raise it and look into the center of your left palm.

There is no special breath. Simply hold the posture and let your heart chant the mantra you love the most. Concentrate on your palm. Carefully gaze at the palm of your hand and meditate on the lines on your palms. Your vision will start enlarging.

At the end, inhale deeply and suspend your breath for a short time, about 10 seconds. Exhale and allow your exhaled breath to purify you and the cosmos. Continue for 11 minutes.

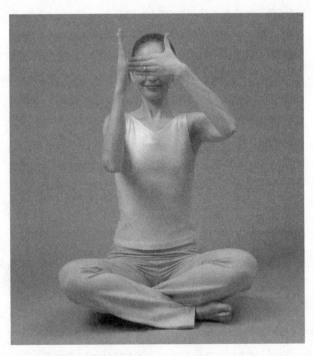

Meditation for Creating Caliber

AFFIRMATION FOR CREATING CALIBER

Yogi Bhajan made the following comments regarding the previous meditation. Read them before you practice it, after you practice, or anytime you wish to inspire your practice.

My love, love me. I'll give you the heavens on earth and you shall play with the earth in the heavens. You and your generations shall be exalted and you shall find peace in your heart. Angels of light shall garland you, and your radiance shall work in every direction. Let your mind be cleansed of karma. Let dharma ignite the light of divinity in and around you. May you live purely and honestly. Let corruption leave you forever. Let your excellence convince people of your commitment. May you win the trust of all and betray none. May you be happy in deed, heart, and soul. Let the purity of heart be your anchor. Let kindness be your shield. Let courage be your gift. May you be peaceful and always under control. Let your commitment exalt you and all who meet you. Let your grace be loved by all and be effective. Let wisdom be your guiding star.

 ## Meditation for Emotional Balance

Practice this meditation when you are worried or upset and you don't know what to do. It is also helpful in those emotional moments when you feel like screaming, yelling, or otherwise misbehaving. Restoring the proper balance of water in your body and slowing your breath rate breaks the pattern of upset and negative emotions and enables you to return to a relaxed state.

Drink a glass of water before practicing this meditation. Sit in Easy Pose. Fold your arms across your chest and lock your hands under your armpits with your palms open and placed against your body. Raise your shoulders up tight against your earlobes, making sure to keep your chin level to the floor. Close your eyes and hold the posture for 3 minutes. Your breath will automatically become slow. As you become accustomed to the meditation, gradually extend your practice time to 11 minutes.

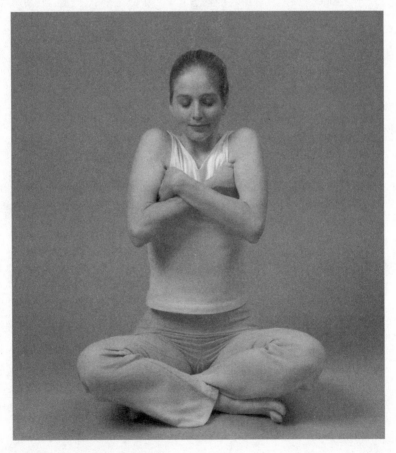

Meditation for Emotional Balance

WORRY IS A MISPLACED PRAYER

 If you find yourself worrying too much, try to reframe your worrisome thoughts into the form of prayers or affirmations. This can help shift negative thought patterns to positive and healing thoughts, which helps reduce stress. For instance, if you are worried about your child at her first day of school, try to change the thought of worry to a prayer or affirmation like "May my daughter have a wonderful day, filled with fun and learning."

Meditation for Mental Control
(Brahm Kalaa)

Brahm Kalaa is another name for Kundalini, your creative life force and your true identity. When you practice this meditation, feel as if you are expanding into the universe. Practice this kriya when you want to turn your dreams into reality. It can help you achieve the victory of self-expression.

Sit in Easy Pose. Cross your arms in front of your chest, and bring your elbows—with a 90-degree bend—parallel to the ground. Place your right palm on top of your left arm, just above the elbow, and the top of your left hand under your right arm, also just above the elbow. Keep your fingers together and straight. Close your eyes and try to stretch your arms out from your shoulders as much as possible. Your breath will become very slow. Continue for 3 minutes. You can gradually increase the time to 11 minutes.

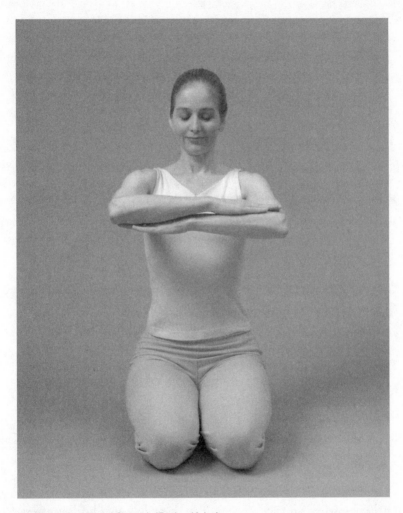

Meditation for Mental Control, (*Brahm Kalaa*)

Meditation for Eliminating Karmas— Letting the Past Be the Past

This meditation can help you let go of the past and heal the negative thoughts associated with your past actions. The hand movements help to strengthen your aura and arc line so you can be present and have a powerful projection.

THE ARC LINE

The arc line—like an energetic halo—circles above the head from ear to ear. Women have an additional arc line that creates another energetic halo effect that shines across her chest, from breast to breast. Both of the female arc lines radiate light. If you could read and interpret that light, you could read your own spiritual identity and destiny. The arc lines become brighter as you hold your identity steady but can become cloudy and broken when you are insecure and compromise your values. Bright arc lines can help shield you from negativity and give you the power of vision and the strength of creating an impact with your presence.

The mantra is both expansive and transforming, helping you to release the past and create a positive future. This meditation can help you when you are grieving. For an even deeper healing effect, try doing this meditation while in a warm bath, scooping a small amount of water over your shoulders as you do the motion of the meditation. The added element of water is soothing to your nervous system and can help you relax intense emotions.

Sit in Easy Pose with a straight spine. Relax your elbows down by your sides, and bring your forearms straight out in front of your body with your palms flat and facing up. Cup your palms slightly and place them a few inches above your knees.

From this relaxed posture begin a repetitive movement of your arms. In a slow, smooth, and graceful motion bring your arms up and back behind your head, making sure to stretch your hands and arms as far back over your shoulders as you can. Imagine you are scooping water and throwing it over your shoulders, with a flick of the wrists. Synchronize the motion of your arms with the chanting of the following mantra:

Wha-hay Guroo, Wha-hay Guroo, Wha-hay Guroo, Wha-hay Jeeo

On each *Wha-hay Guroo*, as well as on the *Wha-hay Jeeo*, do one complete round—scooping up, throwing over your shoulders, and coming back to the starting position, approximately 2 seconds per scoop. The added mantra *Jeeo* represents familiarity, which emphasizes that the experience of your soul is familiar to you, like the familiarity of a close friend. Close your eyes and continue for 3–31 minutes. To end the meditation, inhale, and stretch your hands back as far as possible behind your head. Hold your breath for 10–15 seconds, and then exhale. Repeat this sequence 2 more times and then relax.

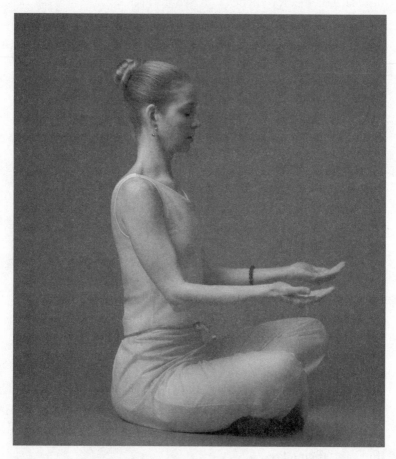

Meditation for Eliminating Karmas—Letting the Past Be the Past, step one

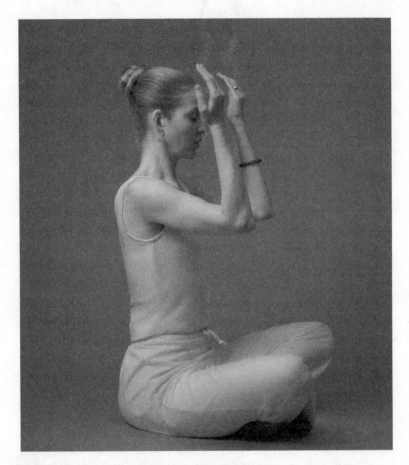

Meditation for Eliminating Karmas—Letting the Past Be the Past, step two

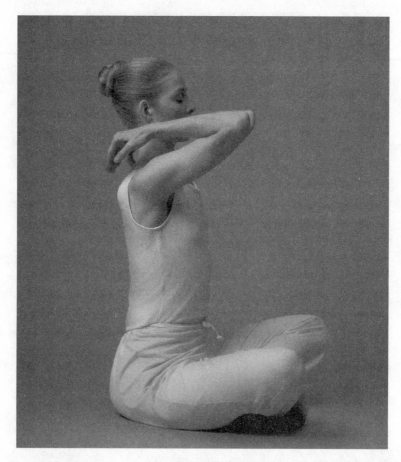

Meditation for Eliminating Karmas—Letting the Past Be the Past, step three

Adi Shakti Mantra:
Tap Your Natural Energy Resources

Chanting this mantra will help you to be less attached to the mind and its fluctuations. It establishes within you an unlimited merger with the Infinite, which is beyond any person and beyond any finite conception. The power of this mantra can be compared to the light of millions and billions of suns. Continued repetition brings a strong healing inner light into your body.

These meditations use the *Adi Shakti Mantra,* a sacred mantra that until recently was never taught to the uninitiated. Yogi Bhajan shared this secret mantra openly when he first began teaching Kundalini Yoga and Meditation in the West in 1969.

Three minutes of practice will give you a taste of its effect. Eleven minutes will clear your mind. Thirty-one minutes will link you to the cosmos and make your best thoughts projective and active. Sixty-two minutes will give you endurance and grace under pressure. Two and a half hours will give you intuition, awaken the Kundalini in order to clear subconscious neuroses and blocks, and open your energy centers to the experience of the inner light and sound of the subtle worlds. Many serious students of Kundalini Yoga do this chant for 2½ hours, before the rise of the sun, for 40 days straight. Chanting for 2½ hours is a commitment. Start slowly. Make sure you relax after chanting this mantra. Walk around a bit or stretch to make sure you are grounded before you begin daily activities again.

The *Adi Shakti Mantra:*

Ek Ong	There is one
Kaar	Creator—Creation

Sat Naam	Truth is the name/identity of that oneness
Siree (*r* pronounced like a soft *d*)	Great is that realization
Wha-hay Guroo	Ecstasy is the result of this realization

Version 1: A Simple Practice

Sit in Easy Pose with a straight spine. Rest your hands over your knees with your fingers in *Gyan Mudra*. Close your eyes to one-tenth open. Chant or listen to the mantra silently or aloud, alone or with a group. This meditation is a key to the unseen cosmos.

Version 2: The Morning Call

Sit in Easy Pose with your hands in *Gyan Mudra* as in Version 1. In this version the mantra is chanted in a 2½-breath cycle as follows:

Start with a deep inhale and chant *Ek Ong Kaar* in one complete exhalation. The *Ek* is very short and chanted as a single sound. As you sound it, pull in your navel point sharply. It will feel like the *Ek* comes from your navel point. The sounds *Ong* and *Kaar* are drawn out and equal in length. When chanted correctly, the sound *Ong* comes through the nose by closing the back of the throat and causing the upper palate to vibrate. *Kaar* resonates from the throat and upper chest.

Inhale deeply again and chant *Sat Naam Siree*. Like the sounding of *Ek, Sat* is a short singular sound generated from the navel point and accompanied by a sharp contraction of this point. *Naam* is a long, drawn-out sound that projects from the chest. *Siree* just escapes your tongue with the last bit of breath that you squeeze out by pulling the navel point in and lifting the diaphragm.

When you chant this mantra, your breath is completely used up during the first two segments of the meditation.

Last, take a short half breath and chant *Wha-hay Guroo*. *Wha* is short and flows off the lips, like the sound of a drop of water hitting a still lake. *Hay* is short and repeated immediately after *Wha* as part of that same word. *Guroo* is medium-long with the *Gu* sound short. It vibrates from the throat and lips. Then begin the cycle again.

 ## Meditation for Fearlessness and Total Support

This meditation can help you feel supported in your life and will help you to reduce attachment to your ego. If you have become numb and withdrawn, this meditation can help create a new sensitivity in you and help you feel supported and connected. The mantra for this meditation is:

Gobinda Gobinda Gobinda Gobinda
Gobinda Gobinda Gobind aah

Gobind means Sustainer. This mantra represents the sustaining energy of the universe. When you chant it, imagine that the earth, the breath you breathe, your body systems, and all other aspects of your life support you. Feel that your own identity is your sustainer.

The rhythm of this mantra in this meditation is specific. Emphasize the first syllable, *Go*. This establishes the breath rhythm.

On the last repetition, notice the short *a,* as in *alive.* The last *aah* is emphasized, as is the first *Go.* The lips must move more than we usually do in English. On *Go,* your lips purse forward slightly, and on *bind,* the corners of your mouth pull back and up. When you have the rhythm correct, it feels like a pleasant lip exercise.

Sit in a comfortable meditative posture with your spine erect and straight. Let your arms relax along your sides. Raise your hands in front of your chest at the level of your heart center. Make fists of both hands. Extend the thumbs. Interlock the thumbs by hooking them and bending them at the first joint. Lock your left thumb over your right thumb (reverse for men). Open your eyelids only one-tenth of the way. Concentrate on the sound of the mantra as you chant and be aware of the Brow Point area. The rhythm of the chant is simple. Chant in a monotone. Inhale and repeat the mantra once. Then inhale a quick breath and begin the mantra again. Continue the chant continuously for 11–31 minutes. To end, inhale deeply and suspend your breath for 30 seconds–1 minute as you keep the thumbs locked. Then relax completely.

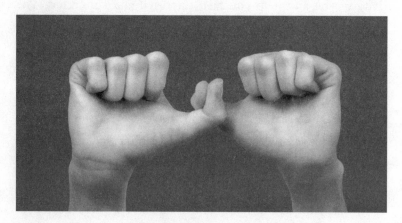

Mudra for Fearlessness and Total Support

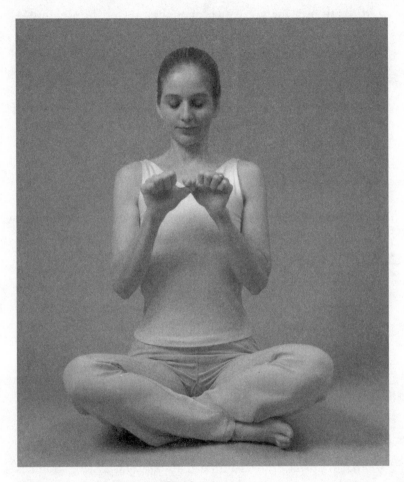

Meditation for Fearlessness and Total Support

Meditation to Bring a Sense of Inner Security

Insecurity comes from not remembering who you are! This meditation uses the same mantra as the previous meditation— *Gobinda*—which means sustainer. Meditating with this mantra will help eliminate insecurity and bring stability to your core identity. Proper repetition of the mantra is tricky. Chant with an exaggerated movement of your lips. Clearly enunciate the *Go* and *d* sounds. The "a" sound is almost silent—like an inflection. Accentuate the first syllable, *Go,* in *Gobinda,* and accentuate all three syllables of *Gobinday.* Each complete repetition lasts about 5 seconds.

Sit in Easy Pose. Your hands are at your heart center (chest level) in Reverse Prayer Pose: the fingers and backs of your hands touch each other back to back, thumbs extending straight out and away from your body. Your eyes look straight ahead, although your eyelids are almost closed.

Part 1:

Meditate and concentrate at the base of your spine. Use your mind to bring energy from the base of your spine to the top of your skull to the tip of your nose. Mentally stretch from the base all the way up the back. Continue to do this with a rhythm, so that your spine moves a little. This part of the meditation has both a physical and a mental effect, and you will break a sweat if it is done correctly. Apply your imagination and concentration with your best and honest intention to eliminate all blocks that are preventing you from healing and realizing your core identity. Continue until you feel that you have cleared any blocks in your spine and your breath is natural. Start by practicing this part of the meditation for just a few minutes.

Part 2:

Now reverse the hands into Prayer Pose, with your palms facing each other and pressed together lightly. The backs of your thumbs are pressed against your chest. Chant the mantra:

Gobinda, Gobinda, Gobinda, Gobinda,
Gobinda, Gobinda, Gobinday

Continue this pattern of mantra repetition in a monotone for 3 to 11 minutes. To end, inhale, exhale, and relax.

Cutting Through Negativity and Darkness, Bringing in Light and Spiritual Identity (*Sodarshan Chakra Kriya*)

This powerful kriya can give you inner happiness and ecstasy, and works effectively to cut through negativity, long-standing neuroses, and low self-esteem. With continued practice, *Sodarschan Chakra Kriya* can help you feel deeply relaxed and strong in even the most challenging situations.

Sodarshan Chakra Kriya uses the mantra *Wha-hay Guroo*. This is the mantra of ecstasy. Generally translated, it means "I am in the presence of wisdom that will bring me from darkness to light."

Sit in a comfortable meditation posture with a straight spine. Focus your eyes on the tip of your nose. Block off your right nostril with your right thumb and inhale slowly and deeply through your left nostril. Suspend your breath and mentally chant the mantra *Wha-hay Guroo* 16 times. Each time you chant a syllable of the mantra, pump your belly in and out (so you're pumping your belly 3 times for each repetition of the mantra, for a total of 48 pumps). Unblock your right nostril and block your left nostril with your right index finger or little finger and exhale powerfully through your right nostril. Continue the sequence by inhaling through your left nostril again.

Sixteen repetitions of the mantra while holding your breath may be difficult for first-time practitioners of this meditation. If you need to let out a breath before all repetitions, simply exhale and begin again. Gradually build your practice to the full 16 repetitions. The recommended times for this meditation are 31 or 62 minutes. Again, this may be too much for beginners. Start slowly with 7–11 minutes, until you feel you are comfortable with the breathing. To finish the meditation, inhale and suspend your breath for 5–10 seconds, and then exhale. Stretch and shake every part of your body for about 1 minute to circulate the energy through your body and to help ground you.

Meditation for the Seventh and Eighth Chakras to Experience Your Expansive Subtle Bodies

You are the spirit, you are the soul, you are the self. You are the honor, you are the source of all sources. You are the redeemer of all redeemers. From you, this creation is born. —YOGI BHAJAN

This simple meditation has a powerful effect on your mind and spirit. When aging challenges you and you doubt your Divine Identity, this is an excellent meditation to do. This meditation also balances your experience of the physical body with a deep experience of your subtle and vast bodies—your true identity of Divine Love.

In this meditation you will be chanting the mantra:

Ang Sung Wha-hay Guroo   Divine Light is in every cell
of my body, every limb of
my body

This mantra is more than a positive affirmation; it is a universal and cosmic statement of your relationship to the Divine.

Sit in Easy Pose with your spine straight. Place your hands in *Gyan Mudra* resting on your knees. Your eyes are focused on the tip of your nose. Chant the mantra *Ang Sung Wha-hay Guroo*. Continue to chant in a relaxed monotone for 3 to 31 minutes. To finish, inhale deeply and suspend your breath as long as possible without straining, and then exhale. Repeat this sequence 2 more times, and then relax.

 Star Meditation

This meditation helps you remember the vastness of your mind and the relationship between you and the cosmos. It helps reduce feelings of depression and leaves you with a feeling of deep relaxation.

Sit in a meditative posture or lie down on the floor or bed. Close your eyes and do the following three-part visualization:

"Feel that you exist. Then turn yourself into a star. This is a very powerful meditation. Feel your body entirely from toe to top. Then feel your body totally as a star—emit the shine. You are turning yourself into a star. Project a lot of light. Then become separate from it and watch it."

Meditation for Intuition and Conquering Fear

This meditation has a special breath pattern that helps you conquer fear and awaken your intuition. As you suspend your breath, you automatically trigger the release of chronic fears (including the fear of death), by creating a Still Point for your mind and body. Practice this meditation to move beyond fear and into your meditative and intuitive mind.

Sit in Easy Pose or in a chair. Relax your elbows by your sides and bring your forearms parallel to the floor and angled out so that they follow the angle of your legs if you are in the cross-legged position. With your palms facing upward, bring the fingertips of each hand together. This is called *Closed Lotus Mudra.* Close your eyes and focus them on your Brow Point. Hold this eye focus. Inhale deeply and exhale. Suspend your breath out as you mentally repeat the mantra sequence *Saa Taa Naa Maa* 4 times. You will be holding your breath out for a total of 16 counts. Inhale deeply, exhale, and begin the sequence again. Continue this sequence with the mental chanting at your brow for 11 minutes. To end, inhale, suspend your breath briefly, and then relax.

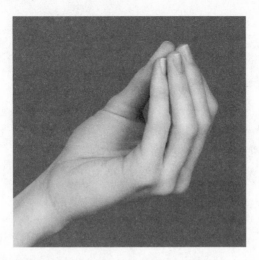

Closed Lotus *Mudra* for Meditation for Intuition
and Conquering Fear

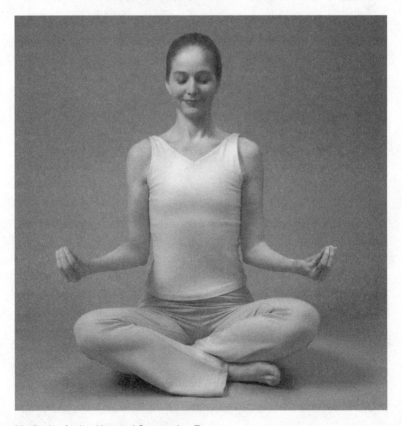

Meditation for Intuition and Conquering Fear

Chanting *Ong* to Remove Fear and Nervousness

Ong is the sound of unity and of manifestation. Chanting this mantra creates a harmony in your physiology and in your thinking, and will remove fear and nervousness from your mind and body.

Sit in a comfortable meditative posture or lie down. Chant the mantra/sound *Ong*. When you chant it, try to vibrate the bones in your skull. You will also feel the vibration in your sinus cavities. After chanting the mantra once, inhale deeply and chant again. Keep trying to find the sound that deeply vibrates within you. Take your time and keep your breath relaxed. It is fine to take several breaths between chanting the mantra.

Meditation to See the Unseen

This meditation will help stimulate your glandular system and your intuition. When you focus your eyes downward toward your chin, you trigger your brain to release emotional stress and enter into a deep state of relaxation. The arm position, although difficult, helps the brain to generate endorphins that give the body endurance and help to strengthen your nervous system. With inner and outer strength, you can hear the subtle voice of your intuition, which is always rooted in your Divine identity. If you practice this meditation daily for 120 days, you will awaken your intuition so you can live through your intuition and not through your fear.

Sit in Easy Pose. Bend your left elbow so that your upper arm is near your ribs and your forearm and hand point upward. Your left palm faces forward with your hand in *Surya Mudra*—the tip of your thumb touching the tip of your ring finger with the other fingers pointing upward. Stretch your right arm straight out and parallel to the ground, keeping your right hand cupped as if you were catching rainwater. Ideally there is no bend in your right elbow. Focus your closed eyes downward and toward the center of your chin. Breathe slowly, deeply, and consciously. Continue for 11 minutes. To finish, inhale and suspend your breath for 15–20 seconds as you stretch your right arm straight while you squeeze all the muscles in your body. Exhale powerfully through your mouth, like a cannon. Repeat this pattern of inhalation, breath suspension, and release 2 more times. Relax.

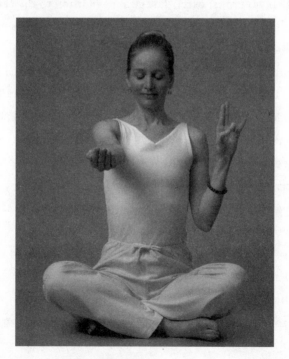

Meditation to See the Unseen

SEE YOUR POWER AS A WOMAN. Touch the heavens and squeeze it to the self and make all the oceans into just a drop. And out of this bring the self into these everlasting pranic winds in which you must squeeze all stars and suns and moons. Beyond that there is a place where you must excel. The gods shall listen to the call of the woman. The sound in the heavens, the murmur of the leaves, the music of the breeze, and sound of the waves, the clouds in the skies, and the dust on the earth, all are in salutation to the call of the woman. The angels, the divines, the sages, the saints are the existence of the very prayer of woman. Calling of woman can penetrate through the heavens and beyond all spaces into the infinity of God, and that's the only power pure enough to manifest God on earth. This is the truth, and you have to experience it.

—YOGI BHAJAN

Resources for Further Growth

Hari Kaur Khalsa

Hari Kaur is available for workshops, classes, yoga, and meditation-for-health lectures and private consultations in person or by phone.

Hari Kaur Khalsa
FDR Station
P.O. Box 7725
New York, NY 10150–7725
www.reachhari.com

3HO Foundation

Founded by Yogi Bhajan, the 3HO Foundation is the teacher-training institution dedicated to Kundalini Yoga as a technique for raising consciousness and expanding awareness.

888-346-2420
www.3HO.org

Kundalini Research Institute (KRI)

KRI was created to establish and preserve the legacy of the teachings of Yogi Bhajan.

kri@3HO.org

International Kundalini Yoga Teachers Association (IKYTA)

The International Kundalini Yoga Teachers Association is a nonprofit professional organization with the mission of training and certifying instructors of Kundalini Yoga, as taught by Yogi Bhajan. Find a Kundalini Yoga teacher in your area from the listing of teachers on this site.

505-753-0423
www.kundaliniyoga.com

YOGA-RELATED PRODUCTS

Ancient Healing Ways

Ancient Healing Ways is an online distributor of Kundalini Yoga–related products, mantras, and healing music; Yogi Bhajan's lecture tapes and CDs; and Yogi Tea and many other health-affirming products.

800-359-2940
www.a-healing.com

Spirit Voyage Music

Spirit Voyage Music is dedicated to the creation and distribution of music for yoga, meditation, and the healing arts.

888-753-4800

www.spiritvoyage.com

Aquarian Times Magazine

Aquarian Times publishes a quarterly magazine dedicated to providing tools to aid individuals in developing a yoga practice, applying new solution-oriented paradigm to problem solving, and developing an expansive, inclusive, and joyous perspective on life.

800-359-2940

www.aquariantimes.com

Yogi Tea Company

www.yogitea.com

FOR FURTHER READINGS ON THE SCIENTIFIC STUDIES OF YOGA AND MEDITATION

The Physical and Psychological Effects of Meditation—A Review of Contemporary Research, by Michael Murphy and Steven Donovan. © 1999–2004 Institute of Noetic Sciences (IONS) www.noetic.org/research/medbiblio.

A Woman's Book of Yoga: Embracing Our Natural Life Cycles, by Machelle M. Seibel, M.D., and Hari Kaur Khalsa (Avery, 2002).

How to Get Smarter, One Breath at a Time, by Lisa Takeuchi Collen, *Time,* January 16, 2006, p. 93.

Suggested Readings on Kundalini Yoga and Meditation

A Woman's Book of Yoga: Embracing Our Natural Life Cycles, by Machelle M. Seibel, M.D., and Hari Kaur Khalsa (Avery, 2002).

The Teachings of Yogi Bhajan, by Yogi Bhajan (KRI, 1977). Notably the transcriptions of Yogi Bhajan's lectures to women 1976–2003, with several years of transcriptions available from Ancient Healing Ways listed above: These notes are a priceless resource of the teachings of Kundalini Yoga and meditation for women.

Videos, DVDs, and Audio Lectures by Yogi Bhajan are also available at Ancient Healing Ways.

The Mind: Its Projections and Multiple Facets, by Yogi Bhajan and Gurucharan Singh Khalsa (KRI, 1999).

The Eight Human Talents—Restore the Balance and Serenity within You with Kundalini Yoga, by Gurmukh (Collins, 2001).

Bountiful, Beautiful, Blissful—Experience the Natural Power of Pregnancy and Birth with Kundalini Yoga and Meditation, by Gurmukh (St. Martin's Press, 2003).

Kundalini Yoga, the Flow of Eternal Power, by Shakti Parwha Kaur Khalsa.

Yoga for Women, by Shakta Kaur Khalsa (KRI, 1996).

Meditation as Medicine: Activate the Power of Your Natural Healing Force, by Dharma Singh Khalsa (Atria, 2001).

Womanheart, by Sangeet Khalsa (Keep Up!, 2002).

Index

About the Author

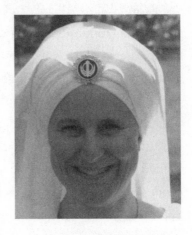

An internationally known Kundalini Yoga teacher and teacher trainer, Hari Kaur Khalsa has studied yoga for more than twenty years. Shortly after her first Kundalini Yoga class, she left her fast-paced, stressful job in the corporate world to pursue a new path and a new job—teaching Kundalini Yoga and meditation. Hari Kaur has been teaching Kundalini Yoga for seventeen years and studied directly with Yogi Bhajan, a world-recognized master of Kundalini Yoga and meditation, working with him as course director of his intensive teacher training program from 1995 until his death in 2004. She continues to train teachers in New York City; Millis, Massachusetts; India; Española, New Mexico, and throughout the world. Hari Kaur has also taught at institutions such as Harvard University, Faulkner Hospital, Newton-Wellesley Hospital Wellness program, all in Massachusetts; the

Omega Institute in New York, and numerous yoga centers, schools, and wellness centers throughout the world. In addition, she has designed and implemented programs for special needs students as well as workout classes for athletes, pregnant women, and the elderly.

Hari Kaur was a founding board member and vice president of the national Yoga Alliance in Clinton, Maryland, an association formulating minimum standards for yoga teachers teaching in the United States. She has also worked with the worldwide Kundalini Research Institute Teacher Trainers Executive Committee, earning her three Community Service Awards, and managed the Newton-Wellesley Hospital yoga program for fifteen years. She now serves as executive representative for the department of information at the United Nations for 3HO, the international Kundalini Yoga non-profit organization founded by Yogi Bhajan and headquartered in Española, New Mexico, focusing on projects with the Commission on the Status of Women and Peace-related issues.

Hari Kaur is a caring, dedicated teacher, and an expert on Kundalini Yoga and meditation. Her knowledge, experience, and down-to-earth interactive style allows all to benefit from this dynamic practice. As a teacher, healer, author, and wife, Hari shares her wisdom, experience, creativity, and love to serve all. She has a natural energy and happiness, a strong grounding and love for life, and a deep meditation practice and realization of the divine here and now.

Hari Kaur has been married for fourteen years to Dave Frank, a world-class jazz musician and composer, who founded the Dave Frank School of Jazz in Manhattan and tours around the world. The two live in New York City.

Hari Kaur's publications include *A Woman's Book of Yoga: Embracing Our Natural Life Cycles,* with Machelle M. Seibel, M.D., published in 2002 by Penguin.

Also available from Hari Kaur Khalsa

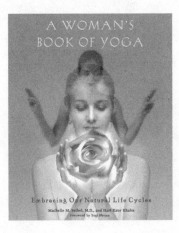

1-58333-137-9

A Woman's Book of Yoga:
Embracing Our Natural Life Cycles

by Machelle M. Seibel, M.D.,
and Hari Kaur Khalsa

Foreword by Yogi Bhajan

Available wherever books are sold

AVERY

a member of Penguingroup (USA) Inc.

www.penguin.com